Optavia Diet Cookbook for Beginners

1000 Days of Delicious Lean and Green Recipes to Help You Keep Healthy and Lose Weight by Harnessing the Power of "Fueling Hacks Meals"

Natrul Frown

© Copyright 2021 Natrul Frown - All Rights Reserved.

In no way is it legal to reproduce, duplicate, or transmit any part of this document by either electronic means or in printed format. Recording of this publication is strictly prohibited, and any storage of this material is not allowed unless with written permission from the publisher. All rights reserved.

The information provided herein is stated to be truthful and consistent, in that any liability, regarding inattention or otherwise, by any usage or abuse of any policies, processes, or directions contained within is the solitary and complete responsibility of the recipient reader. Under no circumstances will any legal liability or blame be held against the publisher for any reparation, damages, or monetary loss due to the information herein, either directly or indirectly.

Respective authors own all copyrights not held by the publisher.

Legal Notice:

This book is copyright protected. This is only for personal use. You cannot amend, distribute, sell, use, quote or paraphrase any part of the content within this book without the consent of the author or copyright owner. Legal action will be pursued if this is breached.

Disclaimer Notice:

Please note the information contained within this document is for educational and entertainment purposes only. Every attempt has been made to provide accurate, up-to-date, and reliable, complete information. No warranties of any kind are expressed or implied. Readers acknowledge that the author is not engaging in the rendering of legal, financial, medical, or professional advice.

By reading this document, the reader agrees that under no circumstances are we responsible for any losses, direct or indirect, which are incurred as a result of the use of information contained within this document, including, but not limited to, errors, omissions, or inaccuracies.

Table of Contents

Introduction 5
Chapter 1: The Basics of Optavia Diet 6
    What is Optavia Diet? 6
    How does the Optavia Diet Plan Work?
    6
    Food to Eat During Optavia Diet 7
    Benefits of Optavia Diet Plan 9
    Tips for Successful Optavia Diet 10
Chapter 2: Lean & Green Recipes 11
    Eggs with Greens 11
    Tomato Basil Egg Cups 12
    Feta Spinach Egg Muffins 13
    Delicious Greek Frittata 14
    Healthy Mushroom Spinach Frittata .. 15
    Easy Egg & Zucchini 16
    Greek Tofu Scramble 17
    Tasty Scrambled Eggs 18
    Kale Egg Cups 19
    Classic Cauliflower Salad 20
    Arugula Cucumber Avocado Salad 21
    Cucumber Tomato Cauliflower Salad 22
    Bell Pepper Soup 23
    Roasted Veggies 24
    Flavorful Skillet Zucchini 25
    Avocado Egg Salad 26
    Nutritious Broccoli Salad 27
    Eggplant Zucchini Stew 28
    Garlic Almonds Cauliflower Rice 29
    Cauliflower Spinach Mash 30
    Basil Cheese Egg Cups 31
    Healthy Eggs Scramble 32
    Smoothie Bowl 33
    Coconut Asparagus Soup 34
    Cauliflower Olive Broccoli Salad 35
    Coconut Broccoli Soup 36
    Cheese Broccoli Salad 37
    Quick Mushroom Soup 38
    Tasty Broccoli Bites 39
    Spinach Mushroom Stir Fry 40
    Lime Garlic Spinach 41
    Pesto Shrimp 42
    Grill Salmon Skewers 43
    Nutritious Salmon Patties 44
    Avocado Tuna Salad 45
    Grilled Salmon Patties 46
    Easy Tuna Cakes 47
    Lemon Pepper Basa 48
    Tuna Patties 49
    Lemon Garlic Shrimp 50
    Baked Halibut 51
    Shrimp & Broccoli 52
    Lemon Garlic Swordfish 53
    Beef Stir Fry 54
    Meatballs 55
    Rosemary Chicken Breast 56
    Asian Chicken Soup 57
    Asparagus Chicken Salad 58
    Turkey Spinach Patties 59
    Meatballs 60
    Chicken Avocado Salad 61
    Chicken Veggie Soup 62
    Avocado Chicken Salad 63
    Chicken Coconut Curry 64
    Kale Chicken Salad 65
    Broccoli Mushroom Stir Fry 66
    Chicken Mushroom Zucchini Stew 67

Turkey Breast with Veggies 68	Easy Strawberry Popsicles 100
Baked White Fish Fillets 69	Chocolate Popsicles 101
Flavorful Catfish Fillets 70	Cinnamon Pumpkin Shake 102
Baked Lemon Cod 71	Choco Almond Butter Drink 103
Creamy Pumpkin Soup 72	Healthy Chia Pudding 104
Cauliflower Pancakes 73	Peanut Butter Coconut Popsicles 105
Tomato Spinach Tofu Scramble 74	Healthy Pumpkin Balls 106
Chicken Egg Muffins 75	Kiwi Popsicles 107
Tomato Spinach Muffins 76	Fluffy Chocó Peanut Butter Mousse 108
Cheese Mint Omelet 77	Chocolate Energy Balls 109
Italian Egg Scrambled 78	Lemon Berry Sorbet 110
Avocado Tuna Salad 79	Avocado Popsicles 111
Salmon Egg Salad 80	Healthy Choco Mousse 112
Healthy Shrimp Salad 81	Cinnamon Pumpkin Ice Cream 113
Tasty Pesto Chicken Salad 82	Lime Blueberry Popsicles 114
Cheese Avocado Shrimp Salad 83	Delicious Brownie Bites 115
Egg Cauliflower Salad 84	Berry Yogurt 116
Chicken Carrot Squash Stew 85	Easy Melon Popsicles 117
Nutritious Fish Stew 86	Raspberry Ice Cream 118
Flavors Zucchini Soup 87	Coconut Lemon Ice Cream 119
Asian Chicken Soup 88	Strawberry Yogurt 120
Greek Cauliflower Rice 89	Berry Frosty 121
Avocado Zucchini Noodles 90	Raspberry Ice Cream 122
Chapter 3: Fueling Recipes 91	Mixed Berry Ice Cream 123
Strawberry Popsicles 91	Almond Milk Ice Bombs 124
Quick Chocolate Mousse 92	Lime Bombs 125
Quick & Easy Brownie 93	Peanut Butter Fat Bombs 126
Silky Chocolate Mousse 94	Quick Strawberry Shake 127
Refreshing Berry Sorbet 95	Mixed Berry Yogurt 128
Energy Balls 96	Chia Berry Coconut Pudding 129
Cashew Butter Bites 97	Chocolate Peppermint Mousse 130
Peanut Butter Energy Balls 98	**Chapter 4: 30-Day Meal Plan** 131
Coconut Blueberry Popsicles 99	**Conclusion** 134

Introduction

The Optavia diet is one of the most popular weight loss diet plans followed by many peoples and celebrities to reduce their excess weight and also maintain healthy body weight. According to U.S News & World report the Optavia diet is ranked in the second position due to its rapid weight loss category. It was a top trending and popular diet plan on Google in 2018. Optavia diet is first introduced and driven by a famous food substitute company Medifast. During the diet period, the company provides you with packaged mini-meals at your doorstep. These mini-meals are known as fuelings which are made up of 24 essential vitamins and nutrients. It also contains probiotics which are also called good bacteria. It helps to improve your digestive system and gut health.

The Optavia diet comes with three Optavia meal plans 5&1 plan, 4&2&1 plan, and 3&3 plan. The first two plans help to reduce your extra weight and the last 3&3 plan helps to maintain healthy body weight. You just need to choose the diet plan as per your health and needs. The plan will execute with fuelings with lean and green meals. The first 5&1 plan contains 5 fuelings with 1 lean and green meal. The Optavia provides full support to their clients to achieve their weight loss goal. It provides a coach to guide and inspire your weight loss journey. The company also provides some additional tools such as a mobile app to set meal reminders and do more tasks using this app.

The cookbook contains Optavia diet recipes written from different categories like lean & green recipes with fueling recipes. All the recipes written in this book are unique and written into easily understandable form with step-by-step instructions. The recipes written in this book are written with their preparation and cooking time. All the recipes end with their nutritional value information. The nutritional value information will help to keep track of daily calorie intake during the Optavia diet. The book also comes with a 30-day meal plan. There are lots of books available in the market on this topic thanks to choosing my book. I hope you love and enjoy all the recipes written in this cookbook.

Chapter 1: The Basics of Optavia Diet

What is Optavia Diet?

The Optavia diet is one of the most popular weight loss programs followed by the peoples who want to reduce their extra weight by replacing their meal. Optavia's diet program was introduced and driven by American nutrition and wellness company Medifast. The Optavia weight loss program is based on eating several types of mini-meal provided by the company in the form of 'Fuelings'. These fuelings are made up of 24 essential vitamins and minerals they are low in calories and high in proteins. The Optavia fuelings contain more than 60 options available. These fuelings food items contain bars, cookies, cereals, puddings, pasta, shakes, soups, and more.

The Optavia food also contains probiotics also known as live microorganisms which come with health benefits. Simply the probiotics are nothing but user-friendly bacteria beneficial for improving digestive health. These user-friendly bacteria are also found in yogurt, probiotics supplements, and fermented foods. The Optavia diet programs suggest taking your lean and green meals with company processed food known as fuelings. If you follow the diet plan properly your body burns fat effectively and helps to reduce your extra body weight. Most of the scientific studies published in different journals indicate that the person who follows Optavia diet plan has noticed significant changes within 8 weeks.

How does the Optavia Diet Plan Work?

The Optavia diet works on three different types of Optavia diet plans. Choose the correct diet plan as per your health and needs. Among these three diet plans, the first two diet plans are used for weight loss purposes, and the last third plan is used to maintain your body weight.

1. Optimal Weight 5&1 Plan

In this plan, you need to consume 6 small meals every day. Out of these 6 meals, 5-nutritionally balanced meals come from Optavia fuelings and 1-meal from a lean and green homemade meal. Most people follow this plan to reduce their extra body weight.

The plan helps you to reduce near about 12 pounds of body weight within 12 weeks.

2. Optimal Weight 4&2&1 Plan

In this plan, you need to consume 7 small meals every day. Out of 7 meals 4 nutritionally balanced small meals come from Optavia fuelings, 2 meals are homemade lean and green meals and 1 is healthy snacks from Optavia fuelings or your own(dairy, starch, and fruit). You have to consume all these meals between two to three hours of gap between each meal.

3. Optimal Weight 3&3 Plan

In this diet plan you have to consume 6 small meals every day. Out of 6 meals 3 nutritionally balanced meals comes from Optavia fuelings, the remaining 3 meals are homemade lean and green meals. You have consumed all these meals between 2 to 3 hours of gap between each meal. This plan is ideal for moderate-weight people to maintain their healthy weight.

The Optavia offers the coach to guide their clients. If you have any doubt or query about the diet plan you can ask your Optavia coach. The company offers additional tools such as mobile apps which help you to keep track of your daily food intake. Using this app you can set your meal reminder and stay connected with the community forums which give you tips that help to lose extra weight and maintain your healthy weight.

Food to Eat During Optavia Diet

The food consumption during the Optavia diet depends on which Optavia plan you have to choose. Most of the foods come in the form of Optavia fuelings. The lean and green meals are homemade meals some healthy snacks are also allowed during the Optavia diet. The Optavia dieters are motivated to choose healthy food items. The types of food allowed during the Optavia diet are mention as follows.

- Fuelings

The Optavia offers more than 60 healthy and nutritious packed fueling in the form of cookies, bars, shakes, brownies, puddings, soups, and more. Consume these fuelings as per your Optavia diet plans. This fueling is made up of 24 essential vitamins and minerals. It is also rich in protein and low in calories. Protein helps to maintain lean muscle mass and repair body cells. The fuelings are also loaded with probiotics which are also called good bacteria help to improve your digestive health.

- Green and non-starchy vegetables

The Optavia diet allows three servings of non-starchy vegetables and two servings of healthy fats. The green and non-starchy vegetables are divided into three subcategories.

Low carb vegetables: Green salads come under this category.

Moderate carb vegetables: Cauliflower and summer squash are moderate carb vegetables.

High Carb Vegetables: Carrots, potatoes, corn, onions, peas, broccoli, and peppers are high-carb foods.

- Lean Meat

The lean meats are low-fat meat. While making lean and green meal 5 to 7-ounce lean protein require with green non-starchy vegetables. The lean meat is divided into three categories.

Lean Meat: Lean meat includes salmon, tuna, herring, farmed catfish, mackerel, lamb, pork chops, etc.

Leaner: Swordfish, halibut, trout, and chicken breast, etc.

Leanest Meat: Shrimp, cod, haddock, tilapia, orange roughy, mahi-mahi, wild catfish, crab, lobster, scallops, etc.

- Use Healthy Fats

Always choose healthy fat options instead of saturated fats during the Optavia diet. It is recommended to choose healthy fats like polyunsaturated fats and monounsaturated fats during the diet. Olive oil, walnut oil, avocado oil, flaxseed oil comes under healthy fat categories. Use healthy fats in the 0 to 2 servings with a green and lean meal.

- Maintain a healthy weight

After reducing the extra weight you have to shift yourself to plan 3&3 to maintain your weight. To maintain ideal body weight add fresh fruit, whole grains, low-fat dairy products, and meatless alternatives into your diet.

Benefits of Optavia Diet Plan

The Optavia diet helps to lose excess body weight and helps to maintain a healthy body weight. The diet comes with various benefits and some of them are mention as follows.

1. Rapid Weight loss

To maintain body weight normal healthy person requires 1600 to 3000 calories per day. The Optavia diet 5&1 program helps to reduce daily calorie consumption at 800 to 1000 calories per day by reducing the portion size. The rapid reduction of calories leads to rapid weight loss. The United States News and World Report ranked Optavia diet at second position for its rapid and fastest weight loss categories.

2. Improve your blood pressure

The intake of low sodium and rapid weight loss during the diet period helps to maintain and improve your blood pressure level. In a 40-week study conducted over 90 peoples who have excess body weight and facing obesity, the Optavia diet plan gives away a significant reduction in blood pressure level.

3. Easy to follow

All the information related to the diet plan are given to its official sites and easy to follow the diet. The diet is mainly based on 3 Optavia diet plans. If your goal is weight loss then the 5&1 or 4&2&1 program is a better option for rapid weight loss. If you are a moderate-weight person and want to maintain your healthy weight then follow the 3&3 diet plan. When you follow the 5&1 plan you only need to prepare 1 green and lean meal daily.

4. Offers Convenience

Most of the diet is depends on packaged foods. You just need to choose the diet plan as per your needs. The company will provide soups, shakes, bars, cookies, puddings, and more at your doorstep. You just need to prepare green and lean meals at your home. You can also order a green and lean meal at your doorstep if you don't have time to prepare at home. The diet not only offers healthy meals at your doorstep but also saves your time and energy.

5. Offers ongoing support

If you facing any difficulty or having any query about diet. You can directly ask your Optavia coach which is available to guide you throughout the year. The coaches not only give you proper guidance but also inspire you to achieve your weight loss goal.

Tips for Successful Optavia Diet

The success of the Optavia diet depends on how you follow the diet plan. The following tips and tricks will help and guide you to achieve your weight loss goal.

1. Use a healthy cooking method while making your green and lean meal. The healthy cooking method includes air frying, broiling, baking, grilling, and more. Do not deep fry your food it may add bad fats to your food and raise calories.
2. When you are following the Optavia diet than always check the portion size of your meal after it is cooked. The right portion size will help you to achieve your goal.
3. Always choose healthy foods which are high in protein and low in calories. Fish like salmon, mackerel, trout, and herrings are a rich source of omega-3 fatty acids. The omega-3 fatty acids help to reduce inflammation and also reduce the risk of heart-related disease.
4. Follow your diet strictly if you are dining out then order healthy and nutritious foods only.
5. Completely avoid alcohol consumption during the diet period it increases your calories, dehydrates your body and increases carbohydrates level, and kicks you out from the fat burning process.
6. If your goal is rapid weight loss then you must do the exercise during the diet period. Regular exercise will improve the metabolic process and helps to lose your bodyweight rapidly.

Chapter 2: Lean & Green Recipes

Eggs with Greens

Preparation Time: 10 minutes
Cooking Time: 10 minutes
Serve: 2

Ingredients:

- 4 eggs, lightly beaten
- 1 cup fresh spinach
- 2 cups chard, stemmed & chopped
- 1 tbsp olive oil
- 1/2 cup cheddar cheese, shredded
- 1 tsp garlic, minced
- 1/2 cup arugula
- Pepper
- Salt

Directions:

1. Heat oil in a pan over medium-high heat.
2. Add arugula, spinach, and chard and sauté for 3 minutes.
3. Add garlic and sauté for 1 minute.
4. In a bowl, whisk eggs with cheese and pour over the veggie mixture.
5. Cover and cook for 5-7 minutes. Season with pepper and salt.
6. Serve and enjoy.

Nutritional Value (Amount per Serving):

- Calories 314
- Fat 25.3 g
- Carbohydrates 3.6 g
- Sugar 1.4 g
- Protein 19.4 g
- Cholesterol 357 mg

Tomato Basil Egg Cups

Preparation Time: 10 minutes
Cooking Time: 20 minutes
Serve: 6

Ingredients:

- 6 eggs
- 1/3 cup sun-dried tomatoes, chopped
- 3 tbsp fresh basil, chopped
- 1/3 cup feta cheese, crumbled
- 1/4 tsp garlic powder
- Pepper
- Salt

Directions:

1. Preheat the oven to 375 F.
2. Spray muffin pan with cooking spray and set aside.
3. In a bowl, whisk eggs with garlic powder, pepper, and salt. Stir in tomatoes, feta cheese, and basil.
4. Pour egg mixture into the muffin pan and bake for 15-20 minutes.
5. Serve and enjoy.

Nutritional Value (Amount per Serving):

- Calories 87
- Fat 6.2 g
- Carbohydrates 1.2 g
- Sugar 1 g
- Protein 6.9 g
- Cholesterol 171 mg

Feta Spinach Egg Muffins

Preparation Time: 10 minutes
Cooking Time: 25 minutes
Serve: 12

Ingredients:

- 2 cups egg whites
- 2 roasted red peppers, chopped
- 2 cups baby spinach, chopped
- 1/4 cup feta cheese, crumbled
- 10 olives, pitted & chopped
- Pepper
- Salt

Directions:

1. Preheat the oven to 350 F.
2. Spray muffin pan with cooking spray and set aside.
3. In a bowl, whisk egg whites with pepper, and salt. Add feta cheese, olives, red pepper, and spinach and stir well.
4. Pour egg mixture into the prepared muffin pan and bake for 25 minutes.
5. Serve and enjoy.

Nutritional Value (Amount per Serving):

- Calories 38
- Fat 1.2 g
- Carbohydrates 1.6 g
- Sugar 1 g
- Protein 5.1 g
- Cholesterol 3 mg

Delicious Greek Frittata

Preparation Time: 10 minutes
Cooking Time: 20 minutes
Serve: 6

Ingredients:

- 6 eggs
- 1/2 cup frozen spinach, defrosted & drained
- 1/2 tsp garlic powder
- 3/4 tsp oregano
- 1/4 cup feta cheese, crumbled
- 1/4 cup olives, chopped
- 1/2 cup tomatoes, diced
- 1/4 cup almond milk
- Pepper
- Salt

Directions:

1. Preheat the oven to 400 F.
2. Spray a 9-inch pan with cooking spray and set aside.
3. In a bowl, whisk eggs with garlic powder, milk, oregano, pepper, and salt.
4. Add olives, feta, tomatoes, and spinach and stir well.
5. Pour egg mixture into the prepared pan and bake in preheated oven for 20 minutes.
6. Serve and enjoy.

Nutritional Value (Amount per Serving):

- Calories 114
- Fat 8.7 g
- Carbohydrates 2.5 g
- Sugar 1.4 g
- Protein 7 g
- Cholesterol 169 mg

Healthy Mushroom Spinach Frittata

Preparation Time: 10 minutes
Cooking Time: 25 minutes
Serve: 2

Ingredients:

- 5 egg whites
- 2 tbsp mushroom, diced
- 1 tbsp onion, diced
- 2 tbsp tomato, diced
- 1 tbsp olive oil
- 1/4 cup feta cheese, crumbled
- 3 tbsp almond milk
- 1 cup spinach, chopped
- Salt

Directions:

1. Preheat the oven to 450 F.
2. Heat oil in an oven-safe pan over medium heat.
3. Add mushrooms, onion, and tomatoes and sauté for 5 minutes.
4. Add spinach and salt and sauté until spinach is wilted.
5. In a small bowl, whisk egg whites with milk.
6. Pour egg mixture over veggies and cook until egg is 80 percent cooked.
7. Sprinkle with crumbled cheese and bake in preheated oven for 5-10 minutes.
8. Serve and enjoy.

Nutritional Value (Amount per Serving):

- Calories 114
- Fat 8.7 g
- Carbohydrates 2.5 g
- Sugar 1.4 g
- Protein 7 g
- Cholesterol 169 mg

Easy Egg & Zucchini

Preparation Time: 10 minutes
Cooking Time: 15 minutes
Serve: 2

Ingredients:

- 2 eggs
- 2 zucchini, chopped
- 1/4 tsp garlic powder
- 1 1/2 tbsp olive oil
- 1 tsp water
- Pepper
- Salt

Directions:

1. Heat oil in a pan over medium-high heat.
2. Add zucchini and sauté for 10 minutes.
3. In a bowl, whisk eggs with water, garlic powder, pepper, and salt.
4. Pour egg mixture over zucchini and stir to scrambled, about 4-6 minutes.
5. Serve and enjoy.

Nutritional Value (Amount per Serving):

- Calories 186
- Fat 15.2 g
- Carbohydrates 7.2 g
- Sugar 3.8 g
- Protein 8 g
- Cholesterol 164 mg

Greek Tofu Scramble

Preparation Time: 10 minutes
Cooking Time: 15 minutes
Serve: 2

Ingredients:

- 8 oz firm tofu, crumbled
- 1/4 cup olives, halved
- 1/2 cup bell pepper, diced
- 1 tsp garlic, minced
- 1/4 small onion, diced
- 1 tbsp olive oil
- 1/2 fresh lemon juice
- 1/2 cup cherry tomatoes halved
- 1/4 cup fresh basil, chopped
- 1 cup fresh spinach, chopped
- 1 tsp tahini paste
- 2 tbsp Nutritional yeast
- Pepper
- Salt

Directions:

1. In a small bowl, mix tofu, lemon juice, nutritional yeast, tahini, and salt and set aside.
2. Heat oil in a pan over medium heat.
3. Add onion and sauté until softened.
4. Add garlic and bell pepper and sauté for 5 minutes.
5. Add tofu mixture and olives and stir well.
6. Add basil and spinach and stir until spinach is wilted.
7. Remove pan from heat and stir in tomatoes. Season with pepper and salt.
8. Serve and enjoy.

Nutritional Value (Amount per Serving):

- Calories 242
- Fat 15.7 g
- Carbohydrates 5 g
- Sugar 4.4 g
- Protein 16.1 g
- Cholesterol 0 mg

Tasty Scrambled Eggs

Preparation Time: 10 minutes
Cooking Time: 5 minutes
Serve: 2

Ingredients:

- 3 eggs
- 1/2 cup tomato, diced
- 1 tbsp olive oil
- 2 tbsp feta cheese, crumbled
- 1 cup baby spinach
- Pepper
- Salt

Directions:

1. Heat oil in a pan over medium heat.
2. Add spinach and tomatoes and sauté until spinach is wilted.
3. Add eggs and stir to scramble. Add cheese and stir well.
4. Season with pepper and salt.
5. Serve and enjoy.

Nutritional Value (Amount per Serving):

- Calories 191
- Fat 15.7 g
- Carbohydrates 3.2 g
- Sugar 2.1 g
- Protein 10.5 g
- Cholesterol 254 mg

Kale Egg Cups

Preparation Time: 10 minutes
Cooking Time: 30 minutes
Serve: 8

Ingredients:

- 8 eggs
- 3 tbsp olive oil
- 1/2 tsp garlic, minced
- 2 cups kale, chopped
- 1/4 cup feta cheese, crumbled
- 1/2 tsp dried thyme
- 1/4 tsp chili flakes
- Pepper
- Salt

Directions:

1. Preheat the oven to 350 F.
2. Spray muffin pan with cooking spray and set aside.
3. Heat oil in a pan over medium heat.
4. Add garlic and sauté for 30 seconds.
5. Add kale and chili flakes and cook for 2 minutes.
6. In a bowl, whisk eggs with pepper and salt. Add kale and thyme to the egg mixture and stir well.
7. Add crumbled cheese and stir well.
8. Pour egg mixture into the muffin pan and bake for 25-30 minutes.
9. Serve and enjoy.

Nutritional Value (Amount per Serving):

- Calories 129
- Fat 10.6 g
- Carbohydrates 2.4 g
- Sugar 0.5 g
- Protein 6.7 g
- Cholesterol 168 mg

Classic Cauliflower Salad

Preparation Time: 10 minutes
Cooking Time: 10 minutes
Serve: 4

Ingredients:

- 1/2 cauliflower head, grated
- 1 cup parsley, chopped
- 2 tbsp fresh lime juice
- 4 tbsp olive oil
- 3 tbsp fresh mint, chopped
- 1 tomato, chopped
- Pepper
- Salt

Directions:

1. Add all ingredients into the bowl and mix well.
2. Serve and enjoy.

Nutritional Value (Amount per Serving):

- Calories 144
- Fat 14.2 g
- Carbohydrates 5.5 g
- Sugar 1.7 g
- Protein 1.5 g
- Cholesterol 0 mg

Arugula Cucumber Avocado Salad

Preparation Time: 10 minutes
Cooking Time: 5 minutes
Serve: 2

Ingredients:

- 1 cucumber, chopped
- 1 avocado, diced
- 2 tbsp fresh basil leaves, chopped
- 1 cup arugula, chopped
- 2 tomatoes, chopped
- 1 tsp fresh lemon juice
- 1 tbsp olive oil
- 1 bell pepper, chopped
- Pepper
- Salt

Directions:

1. Add all ingredients into the bowl and mix well.
2. Serve immediately and enjoy.

Nutritional Value (Amount per Serving):

- Calories 333
- Fat 27.3 g
- Carbohydrates 23.9 g
- Sugar 9.5 g
- Protein 4.9 g
- Cholesterol 0 mg

Cucumber Tomato Cauliflower Salad

Preparation Time: 10 minutes
Cooking Time: 5 minutes
Serve: 4

Ingredients:

For salad:

- 1 cauliflower head, cut into florets
- 1 cucumber, chopped
- 1 cup onion, chopped
- 1/4 cup parsley, chopped
- 1/4 cup olives
- 2 cups cherry tomatoes, cut in half

For dressing:

- 1 tbsp fresh lime juice
- 1/2 tsp garlic, minced
- 2 tbsp olive oil
- Pepper
- Salt

Directions:

1. Add cauliflower florets into the food processor and process until it looks like rice consistency.
2. Add cauliflower rice in a microwave-safe bowl and microwave for 5 minutes.
3. Add cauliflower rice into a large bowl.
4. Add remaining salad ingredients into the bowl and mix well.
5. Mix together dressing ingredients and pour over salad.
6. Toss well and serve.

Nutritional Value (Amount per Serving):

- Calories 130
- Fat 8.3 g
- Carbohydrates 14.3 g
- Sugar 6.7 g
- Protein 3.2 g
- Cholesterol 0 mg

Bell Pepper Soup

Preparation Time: 10 minutes
Cooking Time: 20 minutes
Serve: 4

Ingredients:

- 6 can roasted red peppers, chopped
- 1 tsp oregano
- 2 tbsp olive oil
- 1 onion, chopped
- 3 cups vegetable stock
- 3 tbsp tomato paste
- 1 tbsp garlic, minced
- Pepper
- Salt

Directions:

1. Heat oil in a pot over medium heat.
2. Add onion and garlic and sauté for 2 minutes.
3. Add tomato paste, roasted pepper, stock, oregano, pepper, and salt, and stir well. Bring to boil.
4. Turn heat to medium-low and simmer for 15 minutes.
5. Remove pot from heat. Puree the soup using a blender until smooth.
6. Serve and enjoy.

Nutritional Value (Amount per Serving):

- Calories 117
- Fat 7.5 g
- Carbohydrates 12.3 g
- Sugar 3.2 g
- Protein 2.7 g
- Cholesterol 0 mg

Roasted Veggies

Preparation Time: 10 minutes
Cooking Time: 6 minutes
Serve: 2

Ingredients:

- 1 cup cauliflower florets
- 1 tbsp olive oil
- 1 bell pepper, cut into chunks
- 1 cup zucchini, chopped
- 1/2 tsp ground cumin
- 1 tsp mint
- 2 garlic cloves
- Pepper
- Salt

Directions:

1. Heat oil in a pan over medium heat.
2. Add vegetables and remaining ingredients and stir well. Cover and cook for 5 minutes.
3. Remove cover and cook for 1 minute more.
4. Stir well and serve.

Nutritional Value (Amount per Serving):

- Calories 108
- Fat 7.5 g
- Carbohydrates 10.4 g
- Sugar 5.2 g
- Protein 2.6 g
- Cholesterol 0 mg

Flavorful Skillet Zucchini

Preparation Time: 10 minutes
Cooking Time: 10 minutes
Serve: 4

Ingredients:

- 1 lb zucchini, chopped
- 2 cups cherry tomatoes, halved
- 1/2 onion, chopped
- 1/2 tsp garlic, minced
- 2 tbsp olive oil
- 6 oz feta cheese, crumbled
- 1 jalapeno, minced
- 1 lime juice
- 2 tbsp fresh cilantro, chopped
- Pepper
- Salt

Directions:

1. Heat oil in a pan over medium heat. Add garlic and sauté for 30 seconds.
2. Add zucchini and onion and sauté for 4-5 minutes.
3. Add tomato and jalapeno and cook for 3-4 minutes.
4. Remove pan from heat. Add cilantro, pepper, and salt and stir well.
5. Add cheese and lime juice and stir well.
6. Serve and enjoy.

Nutritional Value (Amount per Serving):

- Calories 217
- Fat 16.5 g
- Carbohydrates 11.6 g
- Sugar 7 g
- Protein 8.5 g
- Cholesterol 38 mg

Avocado Egg Salad

Preparation Time: 10 minutes
Cooking Time: 10 minutes
Serve: 2

Ingredients:

- 6 eggs, hard-boiled, peel & chopped
- 1/3 cup celery, chopped
- 1 avocado, diced
- 1 tbsp mayonnaise
- 2 tbsp fresh lime juice
- Pepper
- Salt

Directions:

1. Add all ingredients into the bowl and mix well.
2. Serve and enjoy.

Nutritional Value (Amount per Serving):

- Calories 436
- Fat 35.2 g
- Carbohydrates 15.7 g
- Sugar 3 g
- Protein 18.9 g
- Cholesterol 493 mg

Nutritious Broccoli Salad

Preparation Time: 10 minutes
Cooking Time: 5 minutes
Serve: 4

Ingredients:

For salad:

- 1 lb broccoli florets
- 1/4 cup onion, chopped
- 1/3 cup sun-dried tomatoes, chopped
- 1/4 cup almonds, sliced
- 1/4 cup feta cheese, crumbled

For dressing:

- 2 tbsp fresh lemon juice
- 1/4 cup olive oil
- 1/8 tsp chili flakes
- 1/2 tsp Dijon mustard
- 1/2 tsp dried oregano
- 1/2 tsp garlic, minced
- Pepper
- Salt

Directions:

1. Add all salad ingredients into the large bowl and mix well.
2. In a small bowl, mix all dressing ingredients and pour over salad.
3. Toss well and serve.

Nutritional Value (Amount per Serving):

- Calories 215
- Fat 18.1 g
- Carbohydrates 10.9 g
- Sugar 3.4 g
- Protein 6.1 g
- Cholesterol 8 mg

Eggplant Zucchini Stew

Preparation Time: 10 minutes
Cooking Time: 5 minutes
Serve: 4

Ingredients:

- 1 lb eggplant, cut into 1/4-inch cubes
- 1 1/4 lbs zucchini, cut into 1/4-inch cubes
- 2 tsp balsamic vinegar
- 1 cup tomatoes, chopped
- 1 tsp olive oil
- Pepper
- Salt

Directions:

1. Heat oil in a saucepan over medium heat.
2. Add eggplant and zucchini and cook for 3 minutes.
3. Add tomatoes, pepper, and salt and cook for 2 minutes.
4. Add vinegar and stir well.
5. Remove pan from heat.
6. Stir well and serve warm.

Nutritional Value (Amount per Serving):

- Calories 70
- Fat 1.7 g
- Carbohydrates 13.2 g
- Sugar 7 g
- Protein 3.2 g
- Cholesterol 0 mg

Garlic Almonds Cauliflower Rice

Preparation Time: 10 minutes
Cooking Time: 15 minutes
Serve: 4

Ingredients:

- 1 medium cauliflower head, cut into florets
- 1/2 tsp garlic, minced
- 2 tbsp olive oil
- 1/2 cup almonds, sliced & toasted
- 1 tbsp fresh lemon juice
- 1/4 cup parsley, chopped
- Salt

Directions:

1. Add cauliflower florets into the food processor and process until they get rice texture.
2. Squeeze out excess liquid from cauliflower rice.
3. Heat oil in a pan over medium heat.
4. Add garlic and sauté for 30 seconds.
5. Add cauliflower rice and cook for 5-10 minutes or until cauliflower rice is lightly golden brown.
6. Remove pan from heat. Stir in lemon juice, parsley, almonds, and salt.
7. Serve and enjoy.

Nutritional Value (Amount per Serving):

- Calories 167
- Fat 13.1 g
- Carbohydrates 10.6 g
- Sugar 4.1 g
- Protein 5.5 g
- Cholesterol 0 mg

Cauliflower Spinach Mash

Preparation Time: 10 minutes
Cooking Time: 15 minutes
Serve: 6

Ingredients:

- 1 cauliflower head, cut into florets
- 2 tbsp olive oil
- 1/8 tsp garlic powder
- 2 cups baby spinach
- 1 cup onion, diced
- Pepper
- Salt

Directions:

1. Add cauliflower florets into the boiling water and cook until tender.
2. Meanwhile, heat oil in a pan over medium-high heat.
3. Add onions and sauté for 5 minutes.
4. Add spinach and stir well. Remove pan from heat.
5. Drain cauliflower florets and reserve about 1 cup of the cooking water.
6. Add cauliflower florets with water into the food processor and process until getting rice-like texture.
7. Add onion and spinach mixture along with garlic powder, pepper, and salt and process until just combined.
8. Serve warm and enjoy.

Nutritional Value (Amount per Serving):

- Calories 61
- Fat 4.8 g
- Carbohydrates 4.5 g
- Sugar 1.9 g
- Protein 1.4 g
- Cholesterol 0 mg

Basil Cheese Egg Cups

Preparation Time: 10 minutes
Cooking Time: 20 minutes
Serve: 6

Ingredients:

- 6 eggs
- 1/4 cup basil, chopped
- 1/4 tsp Italian seasoning
- 1/3 cup goat cheese, crumbled
- Pepper
- Salt

Directions:

1. Preheat the oven to 375 F.
2. Spray muffin pan with cooking spray and set aside.
3. In a bowl, whisk eggs with Italian seasoning, pepper, and salt. Stir in basil and cheese.
4. Pour egg mixture into the muffin pan and bake for 15-20 minutes.
5. Serve and enjoy.

Nutritional Value (Amount per Serving):

- Calories 71
- Fat 5 g
- Carbohydrates 0.4 g
- Sugar 0.4 g
- Protein 6.1 g
- Cholesterol 165 mg

Healthy Eggs Scramble

Preparation Time: 10 minutes
Cooking Time: 10 minutes
Serve: 2

Ingredients:

- 4 eggs
- 2 tbsp olive oil
- 1/4 tsp garlic powder
- 2 cups baby spinach
- 1/2 onion, sliced
- Pepper
- Salt

Directions:

1. Heat oil in a pan over medium-high heat.
2. Add onion and sauté for 5 minutes.
3. Add spinach and stir until spinach is wilted.
4. In a bowl, whisk eggs with garlic powder, pepper, and salt and pour into the pan. Stir constantly until eggs are set.
5. Serve and enjoy.

Nutritional Value (Amount per Serving):

- Calories 165
- Fat 22.9 g
- Carbohydrates 4.6 g
- Sugar 2.1 g
- Protein 12.3 g
- Cholesterol 327 mg

Smoothie Bowl

Preparation Time: 10 minutes
Cooking Time: 5 minutes
Serve: 1

Ingredients:

- 1 avocado, scoop out the flesh
- 1/2 cup ice cubes
- 1/4 cup water
- 1/4 cup almond milk
- 1/4 tsp liquid stevia
- 1/4 tsp vanilla
- 2 tbsp flax meal

For topping:

- 1/4 cup fresh blueberries
- 1 tbsp coconut flakes, toasted
- 1 tbsp pistachios, crushed

Directions:

1. Add all smoothie ingredients into the blender and blend until smooth.
2. Pour smoothie into the serving bowl and top with coconut flakes, blueberries, and pistachios.
3. Serve immediately and enjoy.

Nutritional Value (Amount per Serving):

- Calories 670
- Fat 62.1 g
- Carbohydrates 31.8 g
- Sugar 7.3 g
- Protein 9.4 g
- Cholesterol 0 mg

Coconut Asparagus Soup

Preparation Time: 10 minutes
Cooking Time: 5 minutes
Serve: 4

Ingredients:

- 12 asparagus stalks, chopped
- 1 tsp garlic, minced
- 1 cup onion, diced
- 14 oz coconut milk
- 1 cup vegetable broth
- 2 tsp olive oil
- Pepper
- Salt

Directions:

1. Heat oil in a saucepan over medium heat.
2. Add asparagus, onion, and garlic and sauté for 2 minutes.
3. Season with pepper and salt.
4. Add broth and bring to boil. Remove pan from heat.
5. Add coconut milk and stir well. Puree the soup using a blender until smooth.
6. Serve and enjoy.

Nutritional Value (Amount per Serving):

- Calories 280
- Fat 26.4 g
- Carbohydrates 10.5 g
- Sugar 5.6 g
- Protein 4.9 g
- Cholesterol 0 mg

Cauliflower Olive Broccoli Salad

Preparation Time: 10 minutes
Cooking Time: 5 minutes
Serve: 5

Ingredients:

For salad:

- 3 cup cauliflower florets
- 1/2 cup feta cheese, crumbled
- 1/4 cup olives, sliced
- 3 cups broccoli florets
- 1 small onion, diced

For dressing:

- 1 garlic clove, minced
- 1/4 tbsp Dijon mustard
- 1/4 cup olive oil
- 2 tbsp balsamic vinegar
- Pepper
- Salt

Directions:

1. Add all salad ingredients into the large bowl and mix well.
2. In a small bowl, mix all dressing ingredients and pour over salad.
3. Stir well and serve.

Nutritional Value (Amount per Serving):

- Calories 176
- Fat 14.3 g
- Carbohydrates 9.5 g
- Sugar 3.6 g
- Protein 5.1 g
- Cholesterol 13 mg

Coconut Broccoli Soup

Preparation Time: 10 minutes
Cooking Time: 15 minutes
Serve: 4

Ingredients:

- 2 lbs broccoli florets, chopped
- 1/2 tsp garlic, chopped
- 1 celery stalk, chopped
- 2 tbsp olive oil
- 14 oz coconut milk
- 4 cups vegetable broth
- 1 onion, chopped
- Pepper
- Salt

Directions:

1. Heat oil in a large pot over medium-high heat.
2. Add celery, onion, and garlic, and sauté until onion soften.
3. Add broccoli, broth, and salt and stir well. Bring to simmer until broccoli is softened.
4. Remove pot from heat. Stir in coconut milk.
5. Puree the soup using a blender until smooth.
6. Season with pepper and salt.
7. Serve and enjoy.

Nutritional Value (Amount per Serving):

- Calories 416
- Fat 32.8 g
- Carbohydrates 24.3 g
- Sugar 9.1 g
- Protein 13.8 g
- Cholesterol 0 mg

Cheese Broccoli Salad

Preparation Time: 10 minutes
Cooking Time: 25 minutes
Serve: 6

Ingredients:

- 6 cups broccoli florets
- 2 tbsp olive oil
- 1/3 cup feta cheese, crumbled
- 1/4 cup pine nuts
- Pepper
- Salt

Directions:

1. Preheat the oven to 425 F.
2. Add broccoli florets, oil, pepper, and salt into the bowl and toss well.
3. Spread broccoli onto the baking sheet and roast for 15 minutes.
4. Add crumbled cheese and pine nuts in broccoli and roast for 10 minutes more.
5. Serve and enjoy.

Nutritional Value (Amount per Serving):

- Calories 131
- Fat 10.6 g
- Carbohydrates 7.1 g
- Sugar 2.1 g
- Protein 4.5 g
- Cholesterol 7 mg

Quick Mushroom Soup

Preparation Time: 10 minutes
Cooking Time: 10 minutes
Serve: 4

Ingredients:

- 3 cups mushrooms
- 1/2 cup onion, chopped
- 2 tbsp olive oil
- 3 cups vegetable stock
- 1 tsp thyme
- 1/2 tsp garlic, minced
- Pepper
- Salt

Directions:

1. Heat oil in a saucepan over medium heat.
2. Add onion and garlic and sauté for 2 minutes.
3. Add mushrooms and sauté for 3 minutes.
4. Add pepper, thyme, stock, and salt. Stir well and cook for 5 minutes.
5. Remove pan from heat. Puree the soup using a blender until smooth.
6. Serve and enjoy.

Nutritional Value (Amount per Serving):

- Calories 83
- Fat 7.3 g
- Carbohydrates 4.1 g
- Sugar 2 g
- Protein 2.2 g
- Cholesterol 0 mg

Tasty Broccoli Bites

Preparation Time: 10 minutes
Cooking Time: 20 minutes
Serve: 3

Ingredients:

- 3 cups broccoli florets
- 2 tbsp olive oil
- For seasoning:
- 1/4 cup nutritional yeast
- 1/4 cup almond flour
- 1/4 tsp cayenne
- 1/4 tsp garlic powder
- Salt

Directions:

1. In a small bowl, mix together all seasoning ingredients.
2. Add broccoli florets, oil, and seasoning mixture into the large bowl and toss well.
3. Preheat the oven to 400 F.
4. Spread broccoli florets on a baking sheet and bake for 20 minutes.
5. Serve and enjoy.

Nutritional Value (Amount per Serving):

- Calories 173
- Fat 11.6 g
- Carbohydrates 12.9 g
- Sugar 1.7 g
- Protein 9.2 g
- Cholesterol 0 mg

Spinach Mushroom Stir Fry

Preparation Time: 10 minutes
Cooking Time: 15 minutes
Serve: 4

Ingredients:

- 10 oz mushrooms, sliced
- 1 tsp coconut aminos
- 6 oz baby spinach
- 1 tbsp olive oil
- 1/2 tsp garlic, minced
- 2 tsp nutritional yeast
- 1 tsp vinegar
- Pepper
- Salt

Directions:

1. Heat oil in a pan over medium heat.
2. Add garlic and sauté for 30 seconds.
3. Add mushrooms and sauté for 10 minutes.
4. Add spinach and sauté until spinach is wilted.
5. Add vinegar, coconut aminos, nutritional yeast, pepper, and salt and stir well and cook for a minute.
6. Serve and enjoy.

Nutritional Value (Amount per Serving):

- Calories 63
- Fat 4 g
- Carbohydrates 5 g
- Sugar 1.4 g
- Protein 4.2 g
- Cholesterol 0 mg

Lime Garlic Spinach

Preparation Time: 10 minutes
Cooking Time: 5 minutes
Serve: 2

Ingredients:

- 10 oz fresh spinach
- 1 tsp garlic, minced
- 1 tbsp olive oil
- 1 tbsp lime juice
- 1 lime zest
- Pepper
- Salt

Directions:

1. Heat oil in a pan over medium heat.
2. Add garlic and sauté for 30 seconds. Add spinach and cook until spinach is wilted.
3. Add lime juice, lime zest, pepper, and salt and stir well and cook for a minute.
4. Serve and enjoy.

Nutritional Value (Amount per Serving):

- Calories 101
- Fat 7.6 g
- Carbohydrates 7.7 g
- Sugar 1 g
- Protein 4.3 g
- Cholesterol 0 mg

Pesto Shrimp

Preparation Time: 10 minutes
Cooking Time: 6 minutes
Serve: 4

Ingredients:

- 1 1/2 lbs shrimp, peeled & deveined
- 1/2 cup basil pesto
- Pepper
- Salt

Directions:

1. Add shrimp, basil pesto, pepper, and salt into the bowl and mix well.
2. Cover and place in the refrigerator for 30 minutes.
3. Thread marinated shrimp onto the soaked wooden skewers.
4. Place shrimp skewers onto the hot grill and cook for 2-3 minutes per side.
5. Serve and enjoy.

Nutritional Value (Amount per Serving):

- Calories 203
- Fat 2.9 g
- Carbohydrates 2.7 g
- Sugar 0 g
- Protein 38.8 g
- Cholesterol 358 mg

Grill Salmon Skewers

Preparation Time: 10 minutes
Cooking Time: 6 minutes
Serve: 4

Ingredients:

- 1 1/2 lbs salmon fillets, cut into 1-inch pieces
- 1 cup cilantro
- 4 garlic cloves
- 1/4 tsp cumin
- 1 cup fresh parsley
- 1/2 cup olive oil
- 1/4 cup red wine vinegar
- Salt

Directions:

1. Add cilantro, oil, vinegar, cumin, parsley, garlic, and salt into the blender and blend until smooth.
2. Pour blended mixture into the large bowl.
3. Add salmon pieces and mix well. Cover and place in the refrigerator for 30 minutes.
4. Thread marinated salmon pieces onto the soaked wooden skewers.
5. Place salmon skewers onto the hot grill and cook for 2-3 minutes per side or until cooked through.
6. Serve and enjoy.

Nutritional Value (Amount per Serving):

- Calories 455
- Fat 35.9 g
- Carbohydrates 2.3 g
- Sugar 0.3 g
- Protein 33.8 g
- Cholesterol 75 mg

Nutritious Salmon Patties

Preparation Time: 10 minutes
Cooking Time: 4 minutes
Serve: 4

Ingredients:

- 1 egg, lightly beaten
- 1 1/2 lbs Alaskan salmon, cut into cubes
- 2 tbsp red chili, diced
- 1/2 tsp garlic, minced
- 1 tbsp fish sauce
- 2 tbsp water
- 1 cup cilantro
- 1/4 cup onion, diced
- Pepper
- Salt

Directions:

1. Add salmon and remaining ingredients into the food processor and process until just combined.
2. Spray pan with cooking spray and heat over medium heat.
3. Make the equal shape of patties from the mixture.
4. Place patties on the hot pan and cook for 2 minutes per side.
5. Serve and enjoy.

Nutritional Value (Amount per Serving):

- Calories 270
- Fat 15.2 g
- Carbohydrates 3.5 g
- Sugar 2.6 g
- Protein 31.9 g
- Cholesterol 111 mg

Avocado Tuna Salad

Preparation Time: 10 minutes
Cooking Time: 5 minutes
Serve: 4

Ingredients:

- 10 oz can tuna, drained & flaked
- 2 avocados, peel & cut into cubes
- 2 tbsp olive oil
- 2 tbsp lime juice
- 1/4 cup fresh parsley, chopped
- 1/2 onion, sliced
- Pepper
- Salt

Directions:

1. Add all ingredients into the bowl and mix until well combined.
2. Serve and enjoy.

Nutritional Value (Amount per Serving):

- Calories 360
- Fat 27.2 g
- Carbohydrates 12 g
- Sugar 1.5 g
- Protein 20.3 g
- Cholesterol 21 mg

Grilled Salmon Patties

Preparation Time: 10 minutes
Cooking Time: 10 minutes
Serve: 6

Ingredients:

- 2 eggs, lightly beaten
- 10 oz can salmon, drain & bone remove
- 1/2 onion, chopped
- 1/3 cup cilantro, chopped
- 1/2 tsp garlic, minced
- 1/2 lemon juice
- 1 tbsp Dijon mustard
- Pepper
- Salt

Directions:

1. Add all ingredients into the bowl and mix until well combined.
2. Make the equal shape of patties from the mixture.
3. Place patties on a hot grill and cook over medium-high heat for 2 minutes per side.
4. Serve and enjoy.

Nutritional Value (Amount per Serving):

- Calories 94
- Fat 4.5 g
- Carbohydrates 1.3 g
- Sugar 0.6 g
- Protein 11.5 g
- Cholesterol 81 mg

Easy Tuna Cakes

Preparation Time: 10 minutes
Cooking Time: 6 minutes
Serve: 4

Ingredients:

- 2 eggs, lightly beaten
- 10 oz can tuna, drained & flaked
- 4 tbsp olive oil
- 1/2 cup parsley, chopped
- 2 tsp garlic, minced
- 2 tbsp Dijon mustard
- Pepper
- Salt

Directions:

1. Add all ingredients except oil into the bowl and mix until well combined.
2. Heat oil in a pan over medium heat.
3. Make the equal shape of patties from the mixture.
4. Place patties in a hot pan and cook until lightly golden brown from both the side, about 3 minutes per side.
5. Serve and enjoy.

Nutritional Value (Amount per Serving):

- Calories 244
- Fat 17.2 g
- Carbohydrates 1.5 g
- Sugar 0.3 g
- Protein 21.5 g
- Cholesterol 103 mg

Lemon Pepper Basa

Preparation Time: 10 minutes
Cooking Time: 12 minutes
Serve: 4

Ingredients:

- 4 basa fish fillets
- 2 tbsp parsley, chopped
- 1/2 tsp garlic powder
- 1/4 tsp lemon pepper seasoning
- 1/4 cup fresh lemon juice
- 8 tsp olive oil
- Pepper
- Salt

Directions:

1. Preheat the oven to 425 F.
2. Place fish fillets in a baking dish and drizzle with oil and lemon juice.
3. Sprinkle remaining ingredients over fish fillets and bake for 12 minutes.
4. Serve and enjoy.

Nutritional Value (Amount per Serving):

- Calories 306
- Fat 21.4 g
- Carbohydrates 5 g
- Sugar 3.2 g
- Protein 24 g
- Cholesterol 0 mg

Tuna Patties

Preparation Time: 10 minutes
Cooking Time: 10 minutes
Serve: 8

Ingredients:

- 1 egg, lightly beaten
- 20 oz can tuna, drained
- 1 tbsp lemon zest
- 2 tbsp dill, chopped
- 1/3 cup almond flour
- 1/4 tsp garlic powder
- 2 tbsp olive oil
- 1 tbsp fresh lemon juice
- Pepper
- Salt

Directions:

1. Add all ingredients except oil into the bowl and mix until well combined.
2. Make the equal shape of patties from the mixture.
3. Heat oil in a pan over medium heat.
4. Place patties on the hot pan and cook for 3-4 minutes per side or until lightly golden brown.
5. Serve and enjoy.

Nutritional Value (Amount per Serving):

- Calories 130
- Fat 5.3 g
- Carbohydrates 1 g
- Sugar 0.2 g
- Protein 19.2 g
- Cholesterol 42 mg

Lemon Garlic Shrimp

Preparation Time: 10 minutes
Cooking Time: 6 minutes
Serve: 4

Ingredients:

- 1 1/2 lbs shrimp, peeled & deveined
- 1 tsp garlic, minced
- 1/4 cup cilantro, chopped
- 1/4 cup parsley, chopped
- 2 tbsp olive oil
- 1 tbsp vinegar
- 2 tsp fresh lemon juice
- 1 tbsp lemon zest
- Pepper
- Salt

Directions:

1. In a bowl, toss shrimp with 1 tablespoon oil, pepper, and salt.
2. Thread shrimp onto the soaked wooden skewers.
3. Place skewers onto the hot grill and cooks over medium heat for 3 minutes on each side.
4. In a small bowl, mix remaining oil, parsley, cilantro, garlic, lemon juice, thyme, lemon zest, and vinegar.
5. Brush shrimp skewers with oil mixture.
6. Serve and enjoy.

Nutritional Value (Amount per Serving):

- Calories 267
- Fat 10 g
- Carbohydrates 3.5 g
- Sugar 0.2 g
- Protein 39 g
- Cholesterol 358 mg

Baked Halibut

Preparation Time: 10 minutes
Cooking Time: 12 minutes
Serve: 4

Ingredients:

- 1 lb halibut fillets
- 1/4 tsp garlic powder
- 1/4 tsp smoked paprika
- 1/4 cup olive oil
- 1 lemon juice
- Pepper
- Salt

Directions:

1. Preheat the oven to 425 F.
2. Place fish fillets in a baking dish.
3. Mix together oil, smoked paprika, garlic powder, pepper, lemon juice, and salt and pour over fish fillets and bake for 12 minutes.
4. Serve and enjoy.

Nutritional Value (Amount per Serving):

- Calories 238
- Fat 15.4 g
- Carbohydrates 0.5 g
- Sugar 0.3 g
- Protein 24 g
- Cholesterol 36 mg

Shrimp & Broccoli

Preparation Time: 10 minutes
Cooking Time: 15 minutes
Serve: 2

Ingredients:

- 2 cups broccoli florets
- 1 lb shrimp, peeled & deveined
- 1 tsp Italian seasoning
- 1 tbsp garlic, minced
- 2 tbsp olive oil
- 1/2 fresh lemon juice
- 2 tbsp vegetable stock
- Pepper
- Salt

Directions:

1. Preheat the oven to 425 F.
2. Add shrimp, broccoli, and remaining ingredients into the large bowl and mix well.
3. Spread shrimp and broccoli mixture onto the baking sheet and bake for 15 minutes.
4. Serve and enjoy.

Nutritional Value (Amount per Serving):

- Calories 443
- Fat 19.1 g
- Carbohydrates 12.3 g
- Sugar 2.7 g
- Protein 55 g
- Cholesterol 479 mg

Lemon Garlic Swordfish

Preparation Time: 10 minutes
Cooking Time: 25 minutes
Serve: 2

Ingredients:

- 1 lb swordfish fillets
- 1 lemon zest
- 1 tsp garlic, minced
- 2 tbsp cilantro, chopped
- 1 tsp sesame oil
- 1 tbsp olive oil
- Pepper
- Salt

Directions:

1. Add fish fillets to the baking dish.
2. Mix together remaining ingredients and pour over fish fillets and allow to marinate for 30 minutes.
3. Preheat the oven to 400 F.
4. Baked marinated fish fillets in preheated oven for 25 minutes.
5. Serve and enjoy.

Nutritional Value (Amount per Serving):

- Calories 442
- Fat 21 g
- Carbohydrates 3.2 g
- Sugar 0.8 g
- Protein 58 g
- Cholesterol 113 mg

Beef Stir Fry

Preparation Time: 10 minutes
Cooking Time: 20 minutes
Serve: 4

Ingredients:

- 1 lb ground beef
- 1/4 tsp garlic powder
- 1/4 tsp chili powder
- 8 oz mushrooms, sliced
- 1 onion, sliced
- Pepper
- Salt

Directions:

1. Add beef to a pan and cook over medium-high heat until beef is browned.
2. Add mushrooms, garlic powder, chili powder, onion, pepper, and salt and stir well and cook for 5-10 minutes.
3. Serve and enjoy.

Nutritional Value (Amount per Serving):

- Calories 235
- Fat 7.3 g
- Carbohydrates 4.7 g
- Sugar 2.2 g
- Protein 2.2 g
- Cholesterol 101 mg

Meatballs

Preparation Time: 10 minutes
Cooking Time: 30 minutes
Serve: 4

Ingredients:

- 1 egg
- 1 lb ground beef
- 1/4 cup onion, diced
- 1/4 cup cilantro, chopped
- 1 tbsp olive oil
- 1 tsp Italian seasoning
- 1 tsp garlic, minced
- Pepper
- Salt

Directions:

1. Heat oil in a pan over medium heat.
2. Add onion and garlic and sauté for 5 minutes.
3. Transfer sautéed onion and garlic to the bowl. Add remaining ingredients to the bowl and mix until well combined.
4. Preheat the oven to 350 F.
5. Make the equal shape of balls from the meat mixture and place them onto the parchment-lined baking sheet.
6. Bake meatballs in preheated oven for 20-25 minutes.
7. Serve and enjoy.

Nutritional Value (Amount per Serving):

- Calories 264
- Fat 12 g
- Carbohydrates 1.2 g
- Sugar 0.5 g
- Protein 35.9 g
- Cholesterol 143 mg

Rosemary Chicken Breast

Preparation Time: 10 minutes
Cooking Time: 30 minutes
Serve: 4

Ingredients:

- 2 chicken breasts, boneless
- 1 tsp dried oregano
- 1 tbsp olive oil
- 3 fresh rosemary sprigs
- 5 garlic cloves
- 1 tbsp lemon juice
- 1 tsp smoked paprika
- Pepper
- Salt

Directions:

1. Add chicken and remaining ingredients into the zip-lock bag. Seal bag and place in the fridge for 30 minutes.
2. Preheat the oven to 425 F.
3. Place marinated chicken on a baking sheet and bake for 15 minutes.
4. Flip chicken and cook for 15 minutes more.
5. Serve and enjoy.

Nutritional Value (Amount per Serving):

- Calories 181
- Fat 9.2 g
- Carbohydrates 2.5 g
- Sugar 0.2 g
- Protein 21.6 g
- Cholesterol 65 mg

Asian Chicken Soup

Preparation Time: 10 minutes
Cooking Time: 25 minutes
Serve: 6

Ingredients:

- 1 lb chicken breast, boneless
- 2 tbsp cilantro, chopped
- 2 tsp ginger, minced
- 1 1/2 cups chicken broth
- 8 mushrooms, sliced
- 14 oz coconut milk
- 1/3 cup water
- 1 tbsp curry paste
- 2 tbsp lemongrass, chopped
- 1 tsp salt

Directions:

1. Spray pan with cooking spray and heat over medium heat.
2. Add chicken, curry paste, and ginger to the pan and cook until the chicken is completely cooked.
3. Once the chicken is cooked then add water and simmer for 5 minutes.
4. Remove pan from heat and set aside to cool.
5. Add mushrooms, cilantro, broth, coconut milk, and salt in a large pot and heat over medium heat for 20 minutes.
6. Shred chicken using a fork and add into the pot.
7. Stir and serve.

Nutritional Value (Amount per Serving):

- Calories 274
- Fat 19.6 g
- Carbohydrates 6.2 g
- Sugar 2.8 g
- Protein 19.7 g
- Cholesterol 48 mg

Asparagus Chicken Salad

Preparation Time: 10 minutes
Cooking Time: 10 minutes
Serve: 4

Ingredients:

- 1 lb chicken, cooked & cut into chunks
- 1 1/2 lbs asparagus, cut into 1-inch pieces
- 1 tbsp dill, chopped
- 1 tbsp shallots, minced
- 2 avocados, peel & chopped
- 4 tbsp olive oil
- 3 tbsp lemon juice
- 1 tsp Dijon mustard
- Pepper
- Salt

Directions:

1. Add asparagus into the boiling water and cook until tender, about 5 minutes.
2. Drain asparagus and place into the large bowl.
3. Add remaining ingredients into the bowl and mix well.
4. Serve and enjoy.

Nutritional Value (Amount per Serving):

- Calories 538
- Fat 37.4 g
- Carbohydrates 16.4 g
- Sugar 4 g
- Protein 38.9 g
- Cholesterol 87 mg

Turkey Spinach Patties

Preparation Time: 10 minutes
Cooking Time: 15 minutes
Serve: 4

Ingredients:

- 1 egg
- 1 lb ground turkey
- 1/4 tsp turmeric
- 2 tbsp olive oil
- 3 cups spinach, chopped
- 1 cup feta cheese, crumbled
- 1/4 tsp dried oregano
- Pepper
- Salt

Directions:

1. Add all ingredients except oil into the bowl and mix until well combined.
2. Heat oil in a pan over medium heat.
3. Make the equal shape of patties from the mixture and place onto the hot pan and cook for 5-7 minutes.
4. Turn patties and cook for 5-7 minutes more.
5. Serve and enjoy.

Nutritional Value (Amount per Serving):

- Calories 402
- Fat 28.6 g
- Carbohydrates 2.6 g
- Sugar 1.7 g
- Protein 38.4 g
- Cholesterol 190 mg

Meatballs

Preparation Time: 10 minutes
Cooking Time: 15 minutes
Serve: 4

Ingredients:

- 1 egg
- 1 lb ground turkey
- 2 tbsp parsley, chopped
- 1/2 cup carrots, chopped
- 1/2 cup kale, chopped
- 1/2 tsp garlic powder
- 1 tbsp coconut flour
- 2 tbsp olive oil
- 1/2 cup broccoli florets, chopped
- Pepper
- Salt

Directions:

1. Preheat the oven to 400 F.
2. Add all ingredients into the bowl and mix until well combined.
3. Make the equal shape of balls from the meat mixture and place them onto the parchment-lined baking sheet.
4. Bake meatballs in preheated oven for 15 minutes.
5. Serve and enjoy.

Nutritional Value (Amount per Serving):

- Calories 313
- Fat 20.8 g
- Carbohydrates 4.7 g
- Sugar 1.1 g
- Protein 33.5 g
- Cholesterol 157 mg

Chicken Avocado Salad

Preparation Time: 10 minutes
Cooking Time: 5 minutes
Serve: 4

Ingredients:

- 2 cups cooked chicken, diced
- 2 avocados, peel & chopped
- 2 tbsp fresh lime juice
- 1/2 cup celery, diced
- 1 green apple, diced
- Pepper
- Salt

Directions:

1. Add 1 avocado and lemon juice in a mixing bowl and mash using a fork.
2. Add remaining ingredients into the bowl and mix well.
3. Serve and enjoy.

Nutritional Value (Amount per Serving):

- Calories 117
- Fat 7.5 g
- Carbohydrates 12.3 g
- Sugar 3.2 g
- Protein 2.7 g
- Cholesterol 0 mg

Chicken Veggie Soup

Preparation Time: 10 minutes
Cooking Time: 25 minutes
Serve: 5

Ingredients:

- 1 lb chicken breasts, boneless & skinless
- 3 celery, chopped
- 3 medium carrots, peel & slice
- 1 onion, chopped
- 1 tbsp olive oil
- 5 cups chicken stock
- 2 cups cauliflower rice
- 1 tsp garlic, minced
- Pepper
- Salt

Directions:

1. Heat oil in a large pot over medium heat.
2. Add celery, carrots, and onion and cook until onion is softened.
3. Add broth, garlic, chicken, pepper, and salt. Bring to boil.
4. Turn heat to low and simmer for 5-7 minutes or until chicken is completely cooked.
5. Remove chicken from pot and shred using a fork.
6. Add shredded chicken and cauliflower rice into the pot and stir well. Simmer for 5-8 minutes.
7. Serve and enjoy.

Nutritional Value (Amount per Serving):

- Calories 254
- Fat 10.8 g
- Carbohydrates 9.3 g
- Sugar 5.1 g
- Protein 29.1 g
- Cholesterol 81 mg

Avocado Chicken Salad

Preparation Time: 10 minutes
Cooking Time: 5 minutes
Serve: 6

Ingredients:

- 2 cups chicken, cooked & shredded
- 1 tbsp cilantro, chopped
- 1/4 cup onion, diced
- 2 avocados, peel & chopped
- 1 tsp garlic powder
- 2 tsp fresh lemon juice
- 1/2 tsp salt

Directions:

1. Add all ingredients into the bowl and mix well.
2. Serve immediately and enjoy.

Nutritional Value (Amount per Serving):

- Calories 211
- Fat 14.5 g
- Carbohydrates 6.6 g
- Sugar 0.7 g
- Protein 14.9 g
- Cholesterol 36 mg

Chicken Coconut Curry

Preparation Time: 10 minutes
Cooking Time: 20 minutes
Serve: 4

Ingredients:

- 3 chicken breasts, boneless & cut into chunks
- 2 tbsp curry powder
- 4 cups broccoli florets
- 1/2 fresh lemon juice
- 1 tbsp olive oil
- 20 oz coconut milk
- Salt

Directions:

1. Heat olive oil in a saucepan over medium-high heat.
2. Add chicken and broccoli and cook for 2-3 minutes.
3. Add curry powder and salt and cook until chicken is completely cooked for about 8 minutes.
4. Add lemon juice and coconut milk and stir well.
5. Serve and enjoy.

Nutritional Value (Amount per Serving):

- Calories 607
- Fat 46.2 g
- Carbohydrates 15.8 g
- Sugar 6.5 g
- Protein 37.9 g
- Cholesterol 97 mg

Kale Chicken Salad

Preparation Time: 10 minutes
Cooking Time: 5 minutes
Serve: 3

Ingredients:

- 4 cups kale, chopped
- 2 chicken breasts, cooked & chopped
- 1 avocado, chopped
- 1/4 cup feta cheese, crumbled
- 2 tbsp lime juice
- Pepper
- Salt

Directions:

1. Add all ingredients into the bowl and mix well.
2. Serve and enjoy.

Nutritional Value (Amount per Serving):

- Calories 406
- Fat 23 g
- Carbohydrates 18.1 g
- Sugar 1.3 g
- Protein 34 g
- Cholesterol 98 mg

Broccoli Mushroom Stir Fry

Preparation Time: 10 minutes
Cooking Time: 15 minutes
Serve: 4

Ingredients:

- 2 cups broccoli, cut into florets
- 2 cups mushrooms, sliced
- 1 tbsp ginger garlic paste
- 1 small onion, chopped
- 2 tbsp soy sauce
- 2 tbsp vinegar
- 1/4 cup cashews
- 1/2 cup carrot, shredded
- 1/4 cup vegetable broth

Directions:

1. Add broccoli, ginger garlic paste, mushrooms, onion, and broth in a large pan and cook over high heat until broccoli is softened.
2. Add cashews, soy sauce, vinegar, and carrot and stir well and simmer for 2-4 minutes.
3. Serve and enjoy.

Nutritional Value (Amount per Serving):

- Calories 99
- Fat 4.6 g
- Carbohydrates 11.4 g
- Sugar 3.4 g
- Protein 5 g
- Cholesterol 0 mg

Chicken Mushroom Zucchini Stew

Preparation Time: 10 minutes
Cooking Time: 4 hours
Serve: 6

Ingredients:

- 1 1/2 lbs chicken breasts, boneless & cut into chunks
- 1 tsp thyme, dried
- 1 cup chicken broth
- 3 cups zucchini, diced
- 1 onion, diced
- 8 oz mushrooms, sliced
- 5 oz tomato paste
- 1 tbsp garlic, chopped
- 1 cup bell pepper, diced
- 1 tsp basil, dried
- 1 tsp oregano, dried
- Salt

Directions:

1. Add all ingredients into the Crockpot and stir well.
2. Cover and cook on low for 4 hours.
3. Stir well and serve.

Nutritional Value (Amount per Serving):

- Calories 275
- Fat 9.1 g
- Carbohydrates 11.7 g
- Sugar 6.4 g
- Protein 37.1 g
- Cholesterol 101 mg

Turkey Breast with Veggies

Preparation Time: 10 minutes
Cooking Time: 45 minutes
Serve: 4

Ingredients:

- 1 lb turkey breast, cut into 1-inch cubes
- 1 cup mushrooms, cleaned
- 1/2 lb Brussels sprouts, cut in half
- 1 tsp garlic powder
- 2 tbsp olive oil
- Pepper
- Salt

Directions:

1. Preheat the oven to 350 F.
2. In a small bowl, mix oil, garlic powder, pepper, and salt.
3. Place turkey cubes, mushrooms, and Brussels sprouts in a baking dish. Pour oil mixture on top and mix well.
4. Cover baking dish with foil and bake for 45 minutes.
5. Serve and enjoy.

Nutritional Value (Amount per Serving):

- Calories 209
- Fat 9.1 g
- Carbohydrates 11 g
- Sugar 5.7 g
- Protein 22 g
- Cholesterol 49 mg

Baked White Fish Fillets

Preparation Time: 10 minutes
Cooking Time: 12 minutes
Serve: 4

Ingredients:

- 4 white fish fillets
- 3 tbsp olive oil
- 1 tsp cumin
- 1 tsp onion powder
- 1 tsp paprika
- 1/4 tsp cayenne
- 1 tsp oregano
- 1 tsp garlic powder
- Pepper
- Salt

Directions:

1. Preheat the oven to 450 F.
2. Line baking sheet with foil and set aside.
3. Place fish fillets onto the baking sheet and drizzle with oil.
4. In a small bowl, mix cumin, onion powder, paprika, cayenne, oregano, garlic powder, pepper, and salt and rub over fish fillets.
5. Bake fish fillets in preheated oven for 10-12 minutes.
6. Serve and enjoy.

Nutritional Value (Amount per Serving):

- Calories 189
- Fat 11.7 g
- Carbohydrates 1.8 g
- Sugar 0.5 g
- Protein 19.3 g
- Cholesterol 86 mg

Flavorful Catfish Fillets

Preparation Time: 10 minutes
Cooking Time: 15 minutes
Serve: 4

Ingredients:

- 1 lb catfish fillets, cut 1/2-inch thick
- 1 tsp chili flakes
- 2 tsp onion powder
- 1/2 tsp ground cumin
- 1/2 tsp chili powder
- 1 tbsp dried oregano, crushed
- Pepper
- Salt

Directions:

1. Preheat the oven to 350 F.
2. In a small bowl, mix cumin, chili powder, crushed red pepper, onion powder, oregano, pepper, and salt and rub over fish fillets.
3. Place fish fillets in a baking dish and bake for 15 minutes.
4. Serve and enjoy.

Nutritional Value (Amount per Serving):

- Calories 163
- Fat 8.9 g
- Carbohydrates 2 g
- Sugar 0.5 g
- Protein 18 g
- Cholesterol 53 mg

Baked Lemon Cod

Preparation Time: 10 minutes
Cooking Time: 10 minutes
Serve: 2

Ingredients:

- 1 lb cod fillets
- 1/8 tsp cayenne pepper
- 1 tbsp fresh lemon juice
- 1 1/2 tbsp olive oil
- 1/4 tsp salt

Directions:

1. Preheat the oven to 400 F.
2. Place fish fillets in a baking dish.
3. Drizzle with oil and lemon juice and season with cayenne and salt.
4. Bake in preheated oven for 10 minutes.
5. Serve and enjoy.

Nutritional Value (Amount per Serving):

- Calories 274
- Fat 12.6 g
- Carbohydrates 0.2 g
- Sugar 0.2 g
- Protein 40.6 g
- Cholesterol 111 mg

Creamy Pumpkin Soup

Preparation Time: 10 minutes
Cooking Time: 15 minutes
Serve: 1

Ingredients:

- 1/2 cup pumpkin puree
- 1/2 tsp garlic, chopped
- 1 tbsp onion, chopped
- 2 tsp olive oil
- 1/3 cup water
- 1 tsp vegetable bouillon
- 1/4 cup of coconut milk
- 1/4 tsp curry powder
- Pepper
- Salt

Directions:

1. Heat oil in a pan over medium heat.
2. Add garlic, onion, curry powder, pepper, and salt and sauté for 3-5 minutes.
3. Add remaining ingredients and stir well and simmer until heated through.
4. Puree the soup using a blender until smooth.
5. Serve and enjoy.

Nutritional Value (Amount per Serving):

- Calories 268
- Fat 24.1 g
- Carbohydrates 15 g
- Sugar 6.5 g
- Protein 3 g
- Cholesterol 0 mg

Cauliflower Pancakes

Preparation Time: 10 minutes
Cooking Time: 5 minutes
Serve: 1

Ingredients:

- 1 egg
- 1/4 cup cauliflower rice
- 1/2 tbsp onion, diced
- 1 tbsp olive oil
- 1/4 tsp turmeric
- Pepper
- Salt

Directions:

1. Add all ingredients except oil into the bowl and mix until well combined.
2. Heat oil in a pan over medium heat.
3. Take a tablespoon of the cauliflower mixture and pour onto the hot pan and cook for 3-4 minutes.
4. Serve and enjoy.

Nutritional Value (Amount per Serving):

- Calories 196
- Fat 18 g
- Carbohydrates 3 g
- Sugar 1 g
- Protein 6 g
- Cholesterol 165 mg

Tomato Spinach Tofu Scramble

Preparation Time: 10 minutes
Cooking Time: 7 minutes
Serve: 2

Ingredients:

- 1/2 block firm tofu, crumbled
- 1 cup spinach
- 1/4 cup zucchini, chopped
- 1 tbsp olive oil
- 1/4 tsp ground cumin
- 1 tbsp turmeric
- 1 tomato, chopped
- Pepper
- Salt

Directions:

1. Heat oil in a pan over medium heat.
2. Add zucchini, tomato, and spinach and sauté for 2 minutes.
3. Add tofu, cumin, turmeric, pepper, and salt and stir for 5 minutes.
4. Serve and enjoy.

Nutritional Value (Amount per Serving):

- Calories 105
- Fat 8.5 g
- Carbohydrates 5.1 g
- Sugar 1.4 g
- Protein 3.1 g
- Cholesterol 0 mg

Chicken Egg Muffins

Preparation Time: 10 minutes
Cooking Time: 15 minutes
Serve: 12

Ingredients:

- 10 eggs
- 1 cup cooked chicken, chopped
- 1/4 tsp garlic powder
- 1/4 tsp onion powder
- 1/4 tsp chili powder
- Pepper
- Salt

Directions:

1. Preheat the oven to 400 F.
2. Spray a muffin pan with cooking spray and set it aside.
3. In a bowl, whisk eggs with garlic powder, onion powder, chili powder, pepper, and salt.
4. Add remaining ingredients and stir well.
5. Pour egg mixture into the muffin pan and bake for 15 minutes.
6. Serve and enjoy.

Nutritional Value (Amount per Serving):

- Calories 70
- Fat 4 g
- Carbohydrates 0.4 g
- Sugar 0.3 g
- Protein 8 g
- Cholesterol 145 mg

Tomato Spinach Muffins

Preparation Time: 10 minutes
Cooking Time: 20 minutes
Serve: 12

Ingredients:

- 12 eggs
- 4 tbsp water
- 1 cup fresh spinach, chopped
- 1/2 tsp Italian seasoning
- 1 cup tomatoes, chopped
- Pepper
- Salt

Directions:

1. Preheat the oven to 350 F.
2. Spray a muffin pan with cooking spray and set it aside.
3. In a bowl, whisk eggs with water, Italian seasoning, pepper, and salt. Stir in spinach and tomatoes.
4. Pour egg mixture into the prepared muffin pan and bake for 20 minutes.
5. Serve and enjoy.

Nutritional Value (Amount per Serving):

- Calories 65
- Fat 4.5 g
- Carbohydrates 1 g
- Sugar 0.8 g
- Protein 5.7 g
- Cholesterol 164 mg

Cheese Mint Omelet

Preparation Time: 10 minutes
Cooking Time: 5 minutes
Serve: 1

Ingredients:

- 3 eggs
- 1/2 tsp olive oil
- 2 tbsp feta cheese, crumbled
- 1/4 cup fresh mint, chopped
- 2 tbsp coconut milk
- Pepper
- Salt

Directions:

1. In a bowl, whisk eggs with feta cheese, mint, milk, pepper, and salt.
2. Heat oil in a pan over low heat.
3. Pour egg mixture in the pan and cook until eggs are set.
4. Flip omelet and cook for 2 minutes more.
5. Serve and enjoy.

Nutritional Value (Amount per Serving):

- Calories 274
- Fat 20 g
- Carbohydrates 4 g
- Sugar 2 g
- Protein 20 g
- Cholesterol 505 mg

Italian Egg Scrambled

Preparation Time: 10 minutes
Cooking Time: 10 minutes
Serve: 2

Ingredients:

- 4 eggs
- 1 tbsp olive oil
- 1/4 tsp dried oregano
- 1/2 tbsp capers
- 3 olives, sliced
- 1/2 cup cherry tomatoes, sliced
- 2 tbsp green onions, sliced
- 1 bell pepper, diced
- Pepper
- Salt

Directions:

1. Heat oil in a pan over medium heat.
2. Add bell pepper and green onion and cook until pepper is softened.
3. Add tomatoes, capers, and olives, and cook for a minute.
4. Add eggs and stir until eggs are set.
5. Season with oregano, pepper, and salt.
6. Serve and enjoy.

Nutritional Value (Amount per Serving):

- Calories 231
- Fat 17 g
- Carbohydrates 8 g
- Sugar 5 g
- Protein 12 g
- Cholesterol 325 mg

Avocado Tuna Salad

Preparation Time: 10 minutes
Cooking Time: 5 minutes
Serve: 4

Ingredients:

- 3.5 oz can tuna, drained and flaked
- 1/2 cup onion, chopped
- 1/2 cup celery, chopped
- 1/4 cup parmesan cheese, grated
- 1 1/2 tsp garlic powder
- 1 tbsp dill, chopped
- 1 tsp curry powder
- 2 tbsp fresh lemon juice
- 3/4 cup mayonnaise

Directions:

1. Add all ingredients into the bowl and mix until well combined.
2. Serve and enjoy.

Nutritional Value (Amount per Serving):

- Calories 225
- Fat 15.5 g
- Carbohydrates 14.1 g
- Sugar 4.2 g
- Protein 8 g
- Cholesterol 20 mg

Salmon Egg Salad

Preparation Time: 10 minutes
Cooking Time: 5 minutes
Serve: 4

Ingredients:

- 1 egg, hard-boiled, peel and chopped
- 6 oz salmon, drained and remove bones
- 1 tbsp fresh parsley, chopped
- 1/4 tsp paprika
- 1/2 onion, chopped
- 1/4 cup mayonnaise
- 1 tsp Dijon mustard
- 1 tsp fresh lemon juice
- Pepper
- Salt

Directions:

1. Add all ingredients into the bowl and mix until well combined.
2. Season with pepper and salt.
3. Serve and enjoy.

Nutritional Value (Amount per Serving):

- Calories 135
- Fat 8.7 g
- Carbohydrates 5.1 g
- Sugar 1.7 g
- Protein 10 g
- Cholesterol 63 mg

Healthy Shrimp Salad

Preparation Time: 10 minutes
Cooking Time: 10 minutes
Serve: 4

Ingredients:

- 1 lb shrimp, peeled and deveined
- 2 tbsp onion, minced
- 1/2 cup celery, diced
- 1/2 cup mayonnaise
- 1 1/2 tbsp fresh dill, chopped
- 1 tsp Dijon mustard
- 2 tsp fresh lime juice
- Pepper
- Salt

Directions:

1. Add shrimp in boiling water and cook for 2 minutes.
2. Drain shrimp and transfer in a mixing bowl.
3. Add remaining ingredients into the bowl and mix well.
4. Serve and enjoy.

Nutritional Value (Amount per Serving):

- Calories 255
- Fat 11.9 g
- Carbohydrates 10.4 g
- Sugar 2.3 g
- Protein 26.5 g
- Cholesterol 246 mg

Tasty Pesto Chicken Salad

Preparation Time: 10 minutes
Cooking Time: 5 minutes
Serve: 4

Ingredients:

- 2 chicken breasts, cooked and shredded
- 1/2 cup basil pesto
- 2 celery stalks, chopped
- 1/2 cup parmesan cheese, shredded
- 1/4 cup mayonnaise
- Pepper
- Salt

Directions:

1. Add all ingredients into the bowl and mix until well combined.
2. Serve and enjoy.

Nutritional Value (Amount per Serving):

- Calories 235
- Fat 12.8 g
- Carbohydrates 4.3 g
- Sugar 1.1 g
- Protein 25 g
- Cholesterol 77 mg

Cheese Avocado Shrimp Salad

Preparation Time: 10 minutes
Cooking Time: 10 minutes
Serve: 6

Ingredients:

- 1 lb shrimp
- 1/2 cup tomatoes, chopped
- 2 avocados, chopped
- 1 tsp garlic, minced
- 1 tbsp olive oil
- 1 jalapeno pepper, chopped
- 1/4 cup feta cheese, crumbled
- 1 tbsp fresh lemon juice
- Pepper
- Salt

Directions:

1. Heat oil in a pan over medium heat.
2. Add garlic and saute for 30 seconds.
3. Add shrimp and cook for 5-7 minutes. Remove pan from heat and set aside to cool.
4. Add cooked shrimp and remaining ingredients into the bowl and toss well.
5. Serve and enjoy.

Nutritional Value (Amount per Serving):

- Calories 320
- Fat 22 g
- Carbohydrates 8.3 g
- Sugar 1.1 g
- Protein 23.1 g
- Cholesterol 175 mg

Egg Cauliflower Salad

Preparation Time: 10 minutes
Cooking Time: 10 minutes
Serve: 8

Ingredients:

- 10 eggs, hard-boiled, peel and chopped
- 18 oz cauliflower florets, cooked
- 3 tbsp mustard
- 1/4 cup green onions, chopped
- 1 celery stalk, chopped
- 1 cup mayonnaise
- 3 tbsp dill pickle relish
- Pepper
- Salt

Directions:

1. Add mayonnaise, mustard, dill pickle relish, pepper, and salt into the bowl and mix well.
2. Add cauliflower, eggs, celery, and green onions and stir well.
3. Serve and enjoy.

Nutritional Value (Amount per Serving):

- Calories 225
- Fat 16.7 g
- Carbohydrates 10.1 g
- Sugar 5.4 g
- Protein 9.9 g
- Cholesterol 215 mg

Chicken Carrot Squash Stew

Preparation Time: 10 minutes
Cooking Time: 6 hours
Serve: 6

Ingredients:

- 1 lb chicken breasts, boneless
- 3 1/2 cups vegetable broth
- 2 cups butternut squash, cubed
- 1 onion, chopped
- 1 1/2 tbsp sage, minced
- 1 tsp garlic powder
- 1 cup carrots, chopped
- 1 tbsp olive oil
- Pepper
- Salt

Directions:

1. Heat oil in a pan over medium heat.
2. Add onion and saute until softened.
3. Transfer onion to the Crockpot along with remaining ingredients and mix well.
4. Cover and cook on low for 6 hours.
5. Remove chicken from Crockpot and shred using a fork.
6. Add shredded chicken to the Crockpot and stir well.
7. Serve and enjoy.

Nutritional Value (Amount per Serving):

- Calories 224
- Fat 8.9 g
- Carbohydrates 10.2 g
- Sugar 3.2 g
- Protein 25.7 g
- Cholesterol 67 mg

Nutritious Fish Stew

Preparation Time: 10 minutes
Cooking Time: 35 minutes
Serve: 3

Ingredients:

- 4 white fish fillets
- 1/2 tsp paprika
- 1/4 cup olive oil
- 1/4 tsp pepper
- 1 cup of water
- 1 onion, sliced
- 1 tsp salt

Directions:

1. Add oil, paprika, onion, water, pepper, and salt into the saucepan and stir well. Bring to boil over medium-high heat.
2. Turn heat to medium-low and simmer for 15 minutes.
3. Add fish fillets and cook until fish is cooked.
4. Serve and enjoy.

Nutritional Value (Amount per Serving):

- Calories 515
- Fat 32.3 g
- Carbohydrates 3.7 g
- Sugar 1.6 g
- Protein 50.7 g
- Cholesterol 158 mg

Flavors Zucchini Soup

Preparation Time: 10 minutes
Cooking Time: 25 minutes
Serve: 4

Ingredients:

- 5 zucchini, sliced
- 5 cups vegetable stock
- 1/4 tsp paprika
- 8 oz cream cheese, softened
- 1/4 tsp garlic powder
- 1/4 tsp onion powder
- Pepper
- Salt

Directions:

1. Add zucchini, paprika, garlic powder, onion powder, and stock into the pot and bring to boil over high heat.
2. Turn heat to medium-low and simmer for 20 minutes.
3. Add cream cheese and stir until cheese is melted.
4. Puree soup using a blender until smooth. Season with pepper and salt.
5. Serve and enjoy.

Nutritional Value (Amount per Serving):

- Calories 244
- Fat 20.3 g
- Carbohydrates 10.9 g
- Sugar 5.2 g
- Protein 7.7 g
- Cholesterol 62 mg

Asian Chicken Soup

Preparation Time: 10 minutes
Cooking Time: 30 minutes
Serve: 6

Ingredients:

- 4 chicken breasts, cut into chunks
- 1 tbsp coconut aminos
- 2 tbsp chili garlic paste
- 1/4 cup fish sauce
- 1 tbsp fresh basil, chopped
- 1 tsp ground ginger
- 1 oz fresh lime juice
- 14 oz chicken broth
- 14 oz coconut milk
- 28 oz water
- Pepper
- Salt

Directions:

1. Add all ingredients except chicken into the pot and mix well. Bring to boil over medium-high heat.
2. Add chicken and stir well.
3. Turn heat to medium-low and simmer for 30 minutes.
4. Stir well and serve.

Nutritional Value (Amount per Serving):

- Calories 355
- Fat 23.4 g
- Carbohydrates 5.5 g
- Sugar 2.9 g
- Protein 31.7 g
- Cholesterol 87 mg

Greek Cauliflower Rice

Preparation Time: 10 minutes
Cooking Time: 15 minutes
Serve: 4

Ingredients:

- 10 oz cauliflower rice
- 2 tbsp olive oil
- 2 tbsp sun-dried tomatoes, minced
- 2 cups spinach, chopped
- 1/3 cup vegetable broth
- 1 small zucchini, sliced
- 1/2 tsp garlic, minced
- 1 cup mushrooms, sliced
- 1/2 small onion, diced
- 2 tomatoes, diced
- Pepper
- Salt

Directions:

1. Heat oil in a pan over medium heat.
2. Add mushrooms and onion and sauté for 5 minutes. Add garlic and sauté for 30 seconds.
3. Add cauliflower rice, zucchini, tomato, and broth, and mix well.
4. Cover and cook for 5 minutes. Add Spinach and sun-dried tomatoes and cook for 5 minutes.
5. Season with pepper and salt.
6. Serve and enjoy.

Nutritional Value (Amount per Serving):

- Calories 125
- Fat 8.6 g
- Carbohydrates 9.4 g
- Sugar 5 g
- Protein 4.9 g
- Cholesterol 0 mg

Avocado Zucchini Noodles

Preparation Time: 10 minutes
Cooking Time: 10 minutes
Serve: 6

Ingredients:

- 6 large zucchini, spiralized
- 1 tbsp olive oil

For sauce:

- 3 tbsp olive oil
- 2 tbsp fresh lemon juice
- 1/4 cup pine nuts
- 3/4 cup fresh basil leaves
- 2 ripe avocados
- 1/2 tsp sea salt

Directions:

1. Add all sauce ingredients into the blender and blend until smooth.
2. Heat oil in a pan over medium-high heat.
3. Add zucchini noodles to the pan and cook for 2 minutes.
4. Transfer zucchini noodles to the bowls.
5. Pour blended sauce over zucchini noodles and toss well.
6. Season with pepper and salt.
7. Serve and enjoy.

Nutritional Value (Amount per Serving):

- Calories 245
- Sugar 6.3 g
- Fat 19.9 g
- Protein 6.1 g
- Carbohydrates 17.5 g
- Cholesterol 0 mg

Chapter 3: Fueling Recipes

Strawberry Popsicles

Preparation Time: 10 minutes
Cooking Time: 5 minutes
Serve: 8

Ingredients:

- 2 1/2 cups fresh strawberries
- 1/4 tsp vanilla
- 1/2 cup almond milk

Directions:

1. Add strawberries, vanilla, and almond milk into the blender and blend until smooth.
2. Pour blended mixture into the Popsicle molds.
3. Place popsicle molds in the refrigerator until set.
4. Serve and enjoy.

Nutritional Value (Amount per Serving):

- Calories 49
- Fat 3.7 g
- Carbohydrates 4.3 g
- Sugar 2.7 g
- Protein 0.6 g
- Cholesterol 0 mg

Quick Chocolate Mousse

Preparation Time: 10 minutes
Cooking Time: 5 minutes
Serve: 4

Ingredients:

- 1 tbsp almond milk
- 2 avocados, scoop out the flesh
- 1/2 tsp vanilla
- 3 tbsp cocoa powder
- 5 drops liquid stevia

Directions:

1. Add all ingredients into the blender and blend until smooth.
2. Pour blended mixture into the serving glasses.
3. Place mousse glasses in the refrigerator for 2-3 hours.
4. Serve and enjoy.

Nutritional Value (Amount per Serving):

- Calories 224
- Fat 21 g
- Carbohydrates 11.1 g
- Sugar 0.8 g
- Protein 2.7 g
- Cholesterol 0 mg

Quick & Easy Brownie

Preparation Time: 10 minutes
Cooking Time: 20 minutes
Serve: 4

Ingredients:

- 1 scoop vanilla protein powder
- 1/2 tsp vanilla
- 2 tbsp cocoa powder
- 1/2 cup almond butter, melted
- 1 cup banana, mashed
- 4 drops liquid stevia

Directions:

1. Preheat the oven to 350 F.
2. Line baking dish with parchment paper and set aside.
3. Add all ingredients into the blender and blend until smooth.
4. Pour batter into the baking dish and bake in preheated oven for 20 minutes.
5. Slice and serve.

Nutritional Value (Amount per Serving):

- Calories 80
- Fat 2 g
- Carbohydrates 10 g
- Sugar 5.2 g
- Protein 7 g
- Cholesterol 15 mg

Silky Chocolate Mousse

Preparation Time: 5 minutes
Cooking Time: 5 minutes
Serve: 4

Ingredients:

- 1/2 cup cocoa powder
- 4 oz cream cheese
- 6 drops liquid stevia
- 1/2 tsp vanilla
- 1 1/4 cup heavy cream

Directions:

1. Add all ingredients into the blender and blend until smooth.
2. Pour mixture into the serving glasses.
3. Place mousse glasses in the refrigerator for 1-2 hours.
4. Serve and enjoy.

Nutritional Value (Amount per Serving):

- Calories 254
- Fat 24 g
- Carbohydrates 6 g
- Sugar 0.5 g
- Protein 5.1 g
- Cholesterol 80 mg

Refreshing Berry Sorbet

Preparation Time: 5 minutes
Cooking Time: 5 minutes
Serve: 1

Ingredients:

- 1/2 cup fresh strawberries
- 1/2 cup fresh raspberries
- 4 drops liquid stevia
- 1 tsp fresh lime juice

Directions:

1. Add all ingredients into the blender and blend until smooth.
2. Pour into the air-tight container and place in the refrigerator for 3-4 hours.
3. Serve and enjoy.

Nutritional Value (Amount per Serving):

- Calories 54
- Fat 0.7 g
- Carbohydrates 12 g
- Sugar 6 g
- Protein 1.3 g
- Cholesterol 0 mg

Energy Balls

Preparation Time: 10 minutes
Cooking Time: 10 minutes
Serve: 25

Ingredients:

- 1 cup sunflower seeds
- 1 tbsp water
- 6 drops liquid stevia
- 2 oz chocolate, melted

Directions:

1. Add sunflower seeds into the food processor and process until finely ground.
2. Add water, stevia, and chocolate and process until a stiff dough is a form.
3. Make small balls from the mixture and place them onto the parchment-lined baking sheet.
4. Place baking sheet in the refrigerator for 30 minutes.
5. Serve and enjoy.

Nutritional Value (Amount per Serving):

- Calories 25
- Fat 2.1 g
- Carbohydrates 1.1 g
- Sugar 0.1 g
- Protein 0.7 g
- Cholesterol 0 mg

Cashew Butter Bites

Preparation Time: 5 minutes
Cooking Time: 5 minutes
Serve: 12

Ingredients:

- 1 cup cashew butter
- 8 oz cream cheese
- 1/2 tsp vanilla
- 4 drops liquid stevia

Directions:

1. Add all ingredients into the blender and blend until smooth.
2. Pour blended mixture into the mini muffin liners and place in refrigerator until set.
3. Serve and enjoy.

Nutritional Value (Amount per Serving):

- Calories 190
- Fat 17.1 g
- Carbohydrates 6.5 g
- Sugar 0 g
- Protein 5.2 g
- Cholesterol 21 mg

Peanut Butter Energy Balls

Preparation Time: 5 minutes
Cooking Time: 5 minutes
Serve: 12

Ingredients:

- 3/4 cup peanut butter
- 1 1/2 cup almond flour
- 3/4 tsp ground cinnamon
- 3 tbsp Swerve

Directions:

1. Add all ingredients into the bowl and mix until well combined.
2. Cover bowl and place in the refrigerator for 30 minutes.
3. Remove bowl from the refrigerator and make the equal shape of balls from mixture and place on a parchment-lined baking sheet.
4. Serve and enjoy.

Nutritional Value (Amount per Serving):

- Calories 180
- Fat 14.8 g
- Carbohydrates 10.1 g
- Sugar 5.3 g
- Protein 7 g
- Cholesterol 0 mg

Coconut Blueberry Popsicles

Preparation Time: 5 minutes
Cooking Time: 5 minutes
Serve: 4

Ingredients:

- 3 oz fresh blueberries
- 1/2 cup coconut milk
- 1 cup Greek yogurt
- 1 tsp vanilla
- 12 drops liquid stevia

Directions:

1. Add all ingredients into the blender and blend until smooth.
2. Pour blended mixture into the popsicle molds.
3. Place popsicle molds into the refrigerator until set.
4. Serve and enjoy.

Nutritional Value (Amount per Serving):

- Calories 118
- Fat 7.8 g
- Carbohydrates 8.1 g
- Sugar 6.5 g
- Protein 3.5 g
- Cholesterol 3 mg

Easy Strawberry Popsicles

Preparation Time: 5 minutes
Cooking Time: 5 minutes
Serve: 8

Ingredients:

- 1 1/4 cup fresh strawberries
- 1/3 cup Swerve
- 1 1/2 lemon juice
- 1 1/4 cup coconut cream

Directions:

1. Add all ingredients into the blender and blend until smooth.
2. Pour blended mixture into the popsicle molds.
3. Place popsicle molds into the refrigerator until set.
4. Serve and enjoy.

Nutritional Value (Amount per Serving):

- Calories 96
- Fat 9.1 g
- Carbohydrates 4.1 g
- Sugar 2.5 g
- Protein 1.1 g
- Cholesterol 0 mg

Chocolate Popsicles

Preparation Time: 5 minutes
Cooking Time: 5 minutes
Serve: 6

Ingredients:

- 4 oz chocolate, chopped
- 5 drops liquid stevia
- 1 1/2 cup heavy cream

Directions:

1. Add heavy cream in a small saucepan and heat over medium heat until just begins to boil.
2. Remove saucepan from heat.
3. Add chocolate into the heavy cream and stir well and allow to sit for 5 minutes.
4. Add sweetener and stir until chocolate is melted.
5. Pour melted chocolate mixture into the popsicle molds and place into the refrigerator until set.
6. Serve and enjoy.

Nutritional Value (Amount per Serving):

- Calories 294
- Fat 29.9 g
- Carbohydrates 5.6 g
- Sugar 0.2 g
- Protein 2.4 g
- Cholesterol 80 mg

Cinnamon Pumpkin Shake

Preparation Time: 5 minutes
Cooking Time: 5 minutes
Serve: 1

Ingredients:

- 1 cup almond milk
- 1 tsp vanilla
- 2 tbsp heavy cream
- 3 tbsp pumpkin puree
- 4 drops liquid stevia
- 1 tsp cinnamon
- 1/2 tsp pumpkin spice
- 2 oz cream cheese
- 1/2 cup ice

Directions:

1. Add all ingredients into the blender and blend until smooth.
2. Serve immediately and enjoy.

Nutritional Value (Amount per Serving):

- Calories 375
- Fat 34.6 g
- Carbohydrates 11 g
- Sugar 2.3 g
- Protein 6.6 g
- Cholesterol 103 mg

Choco Almond Butter Drink

Preparation Time: 5 minutes
Cooking Time: 5 minutes
Serve: 2

Ingredients:

- 1 tbsp cocoa powder
- 1 tbsp almond butter
- 2 cups hot water
- 1 scoop chocolate protein powder

Directions:

1. Add all ingredients into the blender and blend for 60 seconds.
2. Serve immediately and enjoy.

Nutritional Value (Amount per Serving):

- Calories 85
- Fat 5.3 g
- Carbohydrates 4 g
- Sugar 0.9 g
- Protein 7.2 g
- Cholesterol 10 mg

Healthy Chia Pudding

Preparation Time: 10 minutes
Cooking Time: 10 minutes
Serve: 2

Ingredients:

- 4 tbsp chia seeds
- 1 cup almond milk
- 1/4 tsp vanilla
- 2 drops liquid stevia
- 1/2 cup raspberries

Directions:

1. Add raspberries, stevia, vanilla, and milk in a blender and blend until smooth.
2. Pour blended mixture into the Mason jar. Add chia seeds and stir well.
3. Seal jar with lid and place in the refrigerator for 3 hours.
4. Serve and enjoy.

Nutritional Value (Amount per Serving):

- Calories 360
- Fat 33.4 g
- Carbohydrates 13 g
- Sugar 5.4 g
- Protein 6.2 g
- Cholesterol 0 mg

Peanut Butter Coconut Popsicles

Preparation Time: 10 minutes
Cooking Time: 5 minutes
Serve: 12

Ingredients:

- 1/2 cup peanut butter
- 2 cans coconut milk
- 1 tsp liquid stevia
- 1/4 tsp vanilla

Directions:

1. Add all ingredients into the blender and blend until smooth.
2. Pour blended mixture into the popsicle molds.
3. Place popsicle molds into the refrigerator until set.
4. Serve and enjoy.

Nutritional Value (Amount per Serving):

- Calories 154
- Fat 15 g
- Carbohydrates 4.3 g
- Sugar 2.4 g
- Protein 3.6 g
- Cholesterol 0 mg

Healthy Pumpkin Balls

Preparation Time: 10 minutes
Cooking Time: 5 minutes
Serve: 18

Ingredients:

- 1 cup almond butter
- 6 drops liquid stevia
- 2 tbsp coconut flour
- 2 tbsp pumpkin puree
- 1 tbsp pumpkin pie spice

Directions:

1. In a bowl, mix together almond butter and pumpkin puree until well combined.
2. Add sweetener, pumpkin pie spice, and coconut flour and mix well.
3. Make the equal shape of balls from the mixture and place onto a parchment-lined baking sheet and place in the refrigerator for 1 hour.
4. Serve and enjoy.

Nutritional Value (Amount per Serving):

- Calories 95
- Fat 8.5 g
- Carbohydrates 4.2 g
- Sugar 0.9 g
- Protein 2.4 g
- Cholesterol 0 mg

Kiwi Popsicles

Preparation Time: 5 minutes
Cooking Time: 5 minutes
Serve: 8

Ingredients:

- 4 kiwi, peeled
- 2 bananas, peeled
- 1 cup coconut milk
- Pinch of salt

Directions:

1. Add all ingredients into the blender and blend until smooth.
2. Pour blended mixture into the popsicle molds.
3. Place popsicle molds into the refrigerator until set.
4. Serve and enjoy.

Nutritional Value (Amount per Serving):

- Calories 118
- Fat 7.5 g
- Carbohydrates 14 g
- Sugar 8 g
- Protein 1.4 g
- Cholesterol 0 mg

Fluffy Chocó Peanut Butter Mousse

Preparation Time: 10 minutes

Cooking Time: 5 minutes

Serve: 4

Ingredients:

- 2/3 cup heavy whipping cream
- 3 tbsp peanut butter, smooth
- 1 tbsp cocoa powder
- 3 tbsp Swerve
- 4 oz cream cheese

Directions:

1. Add all ingredients into the blender and blend until smooth & fluffy.
2. Pour blended mixture into the piping bag.
3. Pipe mousse in serving glasses and place in the refrigerator for 20 minutes.
4. Serve and enjoy.

Nutritional Value (Amount per Serving):

- Calories 245
- Fat 23.5 g
- Carbohydrates 5.9 g
- Sugar 1.2 g
- Protein 5.8 g
- Cholesterol 59 mg

Chocolate Energy Balls

Preparation Time: 10 minutes
Cooking Time: 10 minutes
Serve: 10

Ingredients:

- 1/4 cup peanut butter
- 2 tbsp fresh orange juice
- 1 tbsp chia seeds
- 3/4 cup whey protein powder
- 1 tbsp cocoa powder
- 2 tbsp Swerve

Directions:

1. Add all ingredients into the bowl and mix until well combined.
2. Make the equal shape of balls from the mixture and place onto a parchment-lined baking sheet and place in the refrigerator for 2 hours.
3. Serve and enjoy.

Nutritional Value (Amount per Serving):

- Calories 75
- Fat 4.2 g
- Carbohydrates 3.2 g
- Sugar 1.1 g
- Protein 6.7 g
- Cholesterol 14 mg

Lemon Berry Sorbet

Preparation Time: 5 minutes
Cooking Time: 5 minutes
Serve: 2

Ingredients:

- 1/4 cup blackberries
- 1 tsp fresh lemon juice
- 3/4 tsp liquid stevia
- 1/2 cup raspberries
- 1/2 cup strawberries

Directions:

1. Add all ingredients into the blender and blend until smooth.
2. Pour blended mixture into the container and place in the refrigerator for 3 hours.
3. Serve chilled and enjoy.

Nutritional Value (Amount per Serving):

- Calories 35
- Fat 0.4 g
- Carbohydrates 8.2 g
- Sugar 4.1 g
- Protein 0.9 g
- Cholesterol 0 mg

Avocado Popsicles

Preparation Time: 10 minutes
Cooking Time: 10 minutes
Serve: 6

Ingredients:

- 2 avocado, scoop out the flesh
- 1 tsp vanilla
- 1 cup almond milk
- 1 tsp liquid stevia
- 1/2 cup cocoa powder

Directions:

1. Add all ingredients into the blender and blend until smooth.
2. Pour blended mixture into the popsicle molds.
3. Place popsicle molds into the refrigerator until set.
4. Serve and enjoy.

Nutritional Value (Amount per Serving):

- Calories 130
- Fat 12.2 g
- Carbohydrates 7.2 g
- Sugar 1.6 g
- Protein 2.7 g
- Cholesterol 0 mg

Healthy Choco Mousse

Preparation Time: 10 minutes
Cooking Time: 5 minutes
Serve: 4

Ingredients:

- 2 avocados, scoop out the flesh
- 1/2 tsp vanilla
- 3 tbsp almond milk
- 1/4 cup chocolate chips, melted
- 1/4 cup cocoa powder
- Pinch of salt

Directions:

1. Add all ingredients into the blender and blend until smooth.
2. Pour blended mixture into the serving glasses.
3. Place mousse glasses in the refrigerator for 2-3 hours.
4. Serve and enjoy.

Nutritional Value (Amount per Serving):

- Calories 56
- Fat 0.2 g
- Carbohydrates 12.8 g
- Sugar 6.4 g
- Protein 1.8 g
- Cholesterol 0 mg

Cinnamon Pumpkin Ice Cream

Preparation Time: 5 minutes
Cooking Time: 5 minutes
Serve: 5

Ingredients:

- 1/2 cup pumpkin puree
- 2 cups heavy whipping cream
- 1 tbsp vanilla
- 1 tsp ground cinnamon
- 1 1/2 tsp liquid stevia

Directions:

1. Add all ingredients into a blender and blend until smooth.
2. Pour ice cream mixture into an air-tight container. Cover and place in the freezer for 1 hour.
3. Remove ice cream mixture from refrigerator and beat until smooth.
4. Again place in the refrigerator for 2 hours.
5. Serve chilled and enjoy.

Nutritional Value (Amount per Serving):

- Calories 185
- Fat 18 g
- Carbohydrates 4 g
- Sugar 1 g
- Protein 1 g
- Cholesterol 66 mg

Lime Blueberry Popsicles

Preparation Time: 5 minutes
Cooking Time: 5 minutes
Serve: 6

Ingredients:

- 1/4 cup full-fat coconut cream
- 1/3 cup Swerve
- 1 1/2 cups fresh blueberries
- 1/4 cup fresh lime juice

Directions:

1. Add all ingredients into the blender and blend until smooth.
2. Pour blended mixture into the popsicle molds.
3. Place popsicle molds into the refrigerator until set.
4. Serve and enjoy.

Nutritional Value (Amount per Serving):

- Calories 105
- Fat 9.3 g
- Carbohydrates 5.6 g
- Sugar 3.8 g
- Protein 0.4 g
- Cholesterol 0 mg

Delicious Brownie Bites

Preparation Time: 5 minutes
Cooking Time: 10 minutes
Serve: 13

Ingredients:

- 1/4 cup cocoa powder
- 1/2 tsp vanilla
- 1/4 cup monk fruit sweetener
- 3/4 cup pecans, chopped
- 1/4 cup chocolate chips
- 1/2 cup almond butter
- 1/8 tsp pink salt

Directions:

1. Add pecans, sweetener, almond butter, vanilla, cocoa powder, and salt into the food processor and process until just combined.
2. Transfer mixture into the bowl. Add choco chips and mix well.
3. Make the equal shape of balls from the mixture and place onto a parchment-lined baking sheet.
4. Place baking sheet in the refrigerator for 20 minutes.
5. Serve and enjoy.

Nutritional Value (Amount per Serving):

- Calories 105
- Fat 10 g
- Carbohydrates 4 g
- Sugar 1 g
- Protein 2 g
- Cholesterol 0 mg

Berry Yogurt

Preparation Time: 5 minutes
Cooking Time: 5 minutes
Serve: 6

Ingredients:

- 1 cup yogurt
- 1 tsp vanilla
- 4 cups frozen blackberries
- 1 tbsp fresh lime juice

Directions:

1. Add all ingredients into the blender and blend until smooth.
2. Pour blended mixture into the air-tight container. Cover and place in the freezer for 3 hours.
3. Serve and enjoy.

Nutritional Value (Amount per Serving):

- Calories 45
- Fat 0.6 g
- Carbohydrates 7 g
- Sugar 5 g
- Protein 2 g
- Cholesterol 2 mg

Easy Melon Popsicles

Preparation Time: 5 minutes
Cooking Time: 5 minutes
Serve: 4

Ingredients:

- 3 cups melon, chopped
- 2 drops liquid stevia
- 1 tsp fresh lime juice

Directions:

1. Add all ingredients into the blender and blend until smooth.
2. Pour blended mixture into the popsicle molds.
3. Place popsicle molds into the refrigerator until set.
4. Serve and enjoy.

Nutritional Value (Amount per Serving):

- Calories 41
- Fat 0.2 g
- Carbohydrates 9 g
- Sugar 9 g
- Protein 1 g
- Cholesterol 0 mg

Raspberry Ice Cream

Preparation Time: 5 minutes
Cooking Time: 5 minutes
Serve: 2

Ingredients:

- 1 cup frozen raspberries
- 1/2 cup heavy cream
- 1/4 tsp vanilla
- 1/8 tsp liquid stevia

Directions:

1. Add all ingredients into the food processor and process until smooth.
2. Serve immediately and enjoy.

Nutritional Value (Amount per Serving):

- Calories 145
- Fat 11.1 g
- Carbohydrates 10.2 g
- Sugar 4.7 g
- Protein 2 g
- Cholesterol 41 mg

Coconut Lemon Ice Cream

Preparation Time: 5 minutes
Cooking Time: 5 minutes
Serve: 8

Ingredients:

- 4 egg yolks
- 2 tsp lemon zest
- 4 cups full-fat coconut milk
- 1/2 cup fresh lemon juice
- 1 tsp liquid stevia
- Pinch of salt

Directions:

1. Add all ingredients into the blender and blend until smooth.
2. Pour mixture into the ice cream maker and churn according to the ice-cream maker instructions.
3. Pour mixture into the airtight container. Cover and place in refrigerator until set.
4. Serve and enjoy.

Nutritional Value (Amount per Serving):

- Calories 85
- Fat 7.9 g
- Carbohydrates 1.2 g
- Sugar 0.4 g
- Protein 2 g
- Cholesterol 105 mg

Strawberry Yogurt

Preparation Time: 5 minutes
Cooking Time: 5 minutes
Serve: 8

Ingredients:

- 4 cups frozen strawberries
- 1/2 cup Greek yogurt
- 1 tbsp fresh lemon juice
- 1/4 cup Swerve

Directions:

1. Add all ingredients into the blender and blend until smooth and creamy.
2. Serve immediately and enjoy.

Nutritional Value (Amount per Serving):

- Calories 40
- Fat 0.4 g
- Carbohydrates 7.3 g
- Sugar 5.2 g
- Protein 1.8 g
- Cholesterol 1 mg

Berry Frosty

Preparation Time: 5 minutes
Cooking Time: 5 minutes
Serve: 2

Ingredients:

- 1/2 cup frozen strawberries
- 1/2 cup frozen raspberries
- 4 drops liquid stevia
- 1/2 cup heavy whipping cream, chilled

Directions:

1. Add all ingredients into the blender and blend until smooth.
2. Serve immediately and enjoy.

Nutritional Value (Amount per Serving):

- Calories 130
- Fat 11.1 g
- Carbohydrates 7.2 g
- Sugar 3.6 g
- Protein 1 g
- Cholesterol 41 mg

Raspberry Ice Cream

Preparation Time: 5 minutes
Cooking Time: 5 minutes
Serve: 5

Ingredients:

- 2 cups frozen raspberries
- 1/3 cup Swerve
- 1 cup heavy cream
- 1/4 tsp vanilla

Directions:

1. Add heavy cream into the bowl and beat until stiff peaks form.
2. Add raspberries, vanilla, sweetener into the blender and blend until smooth.
3. Pour raspberry mixture into the heavy cream and fold well.
4. Serve immediately and enjoy.

Nutritional Value (Amount per Serving):

- Calories 100
- Fat 8.9 g
- Carbohydrates 4.4 g
- Sugar 1.9 g
- Protein 1 g
- Cholesterol 33 mg

Mixed Berry Ice Cream

Preparation Time: 10 minutes
Cooking Time: 10 minutes
Serve: 6

Ingredients:

- 2/3 cup heavy cream
- 10 oz frozen mixed berries
- 2 tbsp Swerve

Directions:

1. Add heavy cream into the bowl and beat until stiff peaks form.
2. Add berries and swerve into the blender and blend until smooth.
3. Pour raspberry mixture into the heavy cream and fold well.
4. Serve immediately and enjoy.

Nutritional Value (Amount per Serving):

- Calories 74
- Fat 5.1 g
- Carbohydrates 6.8 g
- Sugar 3.4 g
- Protein 0.6 g
- Cholesterol 18 mg

Almond Milk Ice Bombs

Preparation Time: 10 minutes
Cooking Time: 10 minutes
Serve: 8

Ingredients:

- 1 cup almond milk
- 1 tsp vanilla
- 1/4 cup Swerve
- 1 cup heavy cream

Directions:

1. Add all ingredients into the blender and blend until just combined.
2. Pour mixture into the mini silicone muffins molds and place in the refrigerator until set.
3. Serve and enjoy.

Nutritional Value (Amount per Serving):

- Calories 54
- Fat 6 g
- Carbohydrates 0.8 g
- Sugar 0.1 g
- Protein 0.4 g
- Cholesterol 21 mg

Lime Bombs

Preparation Time: 10 minutes
Cooking Time: 10 minutes
Serve: 16

Ingredients:

- 2 cups macadamia nut milk
- 1/2 cup lime juice
- 1/3 cup Swerve
- 2 cups full-fat coconut milk
- 1/2 tsp vanilla

Directions:

1. Add all ingredients into the blender and blend until just combined.
2. Pour blended mixture into the ice cube tray and place in the refrigerator until set.
3. Serve and enjoy.

Nutritional Value (Amount per Serving):

- Calories 40
- Fat 3.3 g
- Carbohydrates 2.9 g
- Sugar 2.4 g
- Protein 0.5 g
- Cholesterol 1 mg

Peanut Butter Fat Bombs

Preparation Time: 10 minutes

Cooking Time: 10 minutes

Serve: 8

Ingredients:

- 2 tbsp peanut butter
- 4 tsp Swerve
- 3/4 cup almond flour

Directions:

1. Add all ingredients into the bowl and mix until well combined.
2. Cover and place in refrigerator until mixture is firm.
3. Make the equal shape of balls from the mixture and serve.

Nutritional Value (Amount per Serving):

- Calories 90
- Fat 7 g
- Carbohydrates 4 g
- Sugar 0.4 g
- Protein 3.3 g
- Cholesterol 0 mg

Quick Strawberry Shake

Preparation Time: 5 minutes
Cooking Time: 5 minutes
Serve: 1

Ingredients:

- 4 strawberries, halved
- 1 cup almond milk
- 1/2 avocado, diced
- 1/2 cup ice cubes
- 2 drops liquid stevia
- 2 almonds

Directions:

1. Add all ingredients into the blender and blend until smooth.
2. Serve and enjoy.

Nutritional Value (Amount per Serving):

- Calories 84
- Fat 6.1 g
- Carbohydrates 7.2 g
- Sugar 2.4 g
- Protein 1.8 g
- Cholesterol 0 mg

Mixed Berry Yogurt

Preparation Time: 10 minutes
Cooking Time: 10 minutes
Serve: 6

Ingredients:

- 1 cup mixed berries
- 1/2 lemon juice
- 1 tsp vanilla
- 1 cup coconut cream
- 2 tbsp erythritol

Directions:

1. In a bowl, whisk together coconut cream, erythritol, lemon juice, and vanilla and place in the refrigerator for 30 minutes.
2. Add berries and coconut cream mixture into the blender and blend until smooth.
3. Transfer blended mixture into the container. Cover and place in the refrigerator for 1-2 hours.
4. Serve and enjoy.

Nutritional Value (Amount per Serving):

- Calories 105
- Fat 9.7 g
- Carbohydrates 5.2 g
- Sugar 3.2 g
- Protein 1.1 g
- Cholesterol 0 mg

Chia Berry Coconut Pudding

Preparation Time: 5 minutes
Cooking Time: 5 minutes
Serve: 2

Ingredients:

- 1/4 cup raspberries
- 1/4 cup strawberries
- 4 tbsp chia seeds
- 1 cup almond milk
- 1/4 tsp vanilla

Directions:

1. Add all ingredients into the blender and blend until smooth.
2. Pour blended mixture into the glass jar. Cover and place in the refrigerator for 2-4 hours.
3. Serve chilled and enjoy.

Nutritional Value (Amount per Serving):

- Calories 165
- Fat 12.9 g
- Carbohydrates 11 g
- Sugar 2.5 g
- Protein 3.3 g
- Cholesterol 0 mg

Chocolate Peppermint Mousse

Preparation Time: 5 minutes
Cooking Time: 5 minutes
Serve: 4

Ingredients:

- 1 1/4 cup heavy cream
- 1/2 cup cocoa powder
- 1/2 tsp peppermint extract
- 5 drop liquid stevia
- 4 oz cream cheese

Directions:

1. Add all ingredients into the blender and blend until smooth.
2. Pour mixture into the serving glasses.
3. Place serving glasses in the refrigerator for 2 hours.
4. Serve and enjoy.

Nutritional Value (Amount per Serving):

- Calories 255
- Fat 25.2 g
- Carbohydrates 7.8 g
- Sugar 0.4 g
- Protein 4.9 g
- Cholesterol 83 mg

Chapter 4: 30-Day Meal Plan

Day 1

Breakfast-Eggs with Greens

Lunch- Cheese Broccoli Salad

Dinner-Lemon Pepper Basa

Day 2

Breakfast-Cauliflower Pancakes

Lunch- Coconut Broccoli Soup

Dinner-Baked Halibut

Day 3

Breakfast-Cheese Mint Omelet

Lunch- Cauliflower Olive Broccoli Salad

Dinner-Lemon Garlic Swordfish

Day 4

Breakfast-Italian Egg Scrambled

Lunch- Coconut Asparagus Soup

Dinner-Rosemary Chicken Breast

Day 5

Breakfast-Tomato Spinach Muffins

Lunch- Cauliflower Spinach Mash

Dinner-Chicken Mushroom Zucchini Stew

Day 6

Breakfast-Basil Cheese Egg Cups

Lunch- Eggplant Zucchini Stew

Dinner-Turkey Breast with Veggies

Day 7

Breakfast-Tomato Spinach Tofu Scramble

Lunch- Nutritious Broccoli Salad

Dinner-Baked Lemon Cod

Day 8

Breakfast-Smoothie Bowl

Lunch- Avocado Egg Salad

Dinner-Flavorful Catfish Fillets

Day 9

Breakfast-Healthy Eggs Scramble

Lunch- Bell Pepper Soup

Dinner-Avocado Tuna Salad

Day 10

Breakfast-Kale Egg Cups

Lunch- Cucumber Tomato Cauliflower Salad

Dinner-Nutritious Fish Stew

Day 11

Breakfast-Healthy Mushroom Spinach Frittata

Lunch- Tasty Scrambled Eggs

Dinner-Greek Cauliflower Rice

Day 12

Breakfast-Delicious Greek Frittata

Lunch- Arugula Cucumber Avocado Salad

Dinner-Avocado Zucchini Noodles

Day 13

Breakfast-Feta Spinach Egg Muffins

Lunch- Classic Cauliflower Salad

Dinner-Garlic Almonds Cauliflower Rice

Day 14

Breakfast-Tomato Basil Egg Cups

Lunch- Greek Tofu Scramble

Dinner-Flavorful Skillet Zucchini

Day 15

Breakfast-Eggs with Greens

Lunch- Easy Egg & Zucchini

Dinner-Roasted Veggies

Day 16

Breakfast-Eggs with Greens

Lunch- Cheese Broccoli Salad

Dinner-Lemon Pepper Basa

Day 17

Breakfast-Cauliflower Pancakes

Lunch- Coconut Broccoli Soup

Dinner-Baked Halibut

Day 18

Breakfast-Cheese Mint Omelet

Lunch- Cauliflower Olive Broccoli Salad

Dinner-Lemon Garlic Swordfish

Day 19

Breakfast-Italian Egg Scrambled

Lunch- Coconut Asparagus Soup

Dinner-Rosemary Chicken Breast

Day 20

Breakfast-Tomato Spinach Muffins

Lunch- Cauliflower Spinach Mash

Dinner-Chicken Mushroom Zucchini Stew

Day 21

Breakfast-Basil Cheese Egg Cups

Lunch- Eggplant Zucchini Stew

Dinner-Turkey Breast with Veggies

Day 22

Breakfast-Tomato Spinach Tofu Scramble

Lunch- Nutritious Broccoli Salad

Dinner-Baked Lemon Cod

Day 23

Breakfast-Smoothie Bowl

Lunch- Avocado Egg Salad

Dinner-Flavorful Catfish Fillets

Day 24

Breakfast-Healthy Eggs Scramble

Lunch- Bell Pepper Soup

Dinner-Avocado Tuna Salad

Day 25

Breakfast-Kale Egg Cups

Lunch- Cucumber Tomato Cauliflower Salad

Dinner-Nutritious Fish Stew

Day 26

Breakfast-Healthy Mushroom Spinach Frittata

Lunch- Tasty Scrambled Eggs

Dinner-Greek Cauliflower Rice

Day 27

Breakfast-Delicious Greek Frittata

Lunch- Arugula Cucumber Avocado Salad

Dinner-Avocado Zucchini Noodles

Day 28

Breakfast-Feta Spinach Egg Muffins

Lunch- Classic Cauliflower Salad

Dinner-Garlic Almonds Cauliflower Rice

Day 29

Breakfast-Tomato Basil Egg Cups

Lunch- Greek Tofu Scramble

Dinner-Flavorful Skillet Zucchini

Day 30

Breakfast-Eggs with Greens

Lunch- Easy Egg & Zucchini

Dinner-Roasted Veggies

Conclusion

The Optavia diet is one of the most popular weight loss diet plans followed by many peoples and celebrities to reduce their excess weight and also maintain healthy body weight. According to U.S News & World report the Optavia diet is ranked in the second position due to its rapid weight loss category. It was a top trending and popular diet plan on Google in 2018. Optavia diet is first introduced and driven by a famous food substitute company Medifast. During the diet period, the company provides you with packaged mini-meals at your doorstep. These mini-meals are known as fuelings which are made up of 24 essential vitamins and nutrients. It also contains probiotics which are also called good bacteria. It helps to improve your digestive system and gut health.

The cookbook contains Optavia diet recipes written from different categories like lean & green recipes with fueling recipes. All the recipes written in this book are unique and written into easily understandable form with step-by-step instructions. The recipes written in this book are written with their preparation and cooking time. All the recipes end with their nutritional value information. The nutritional value information will help to keep track of daily calorie intake during the Optavia diet.

CPSIA information can be obtained
at www.ICGtesting.com
Printed in the USA
BVHW061912220621
610213BV00003B/588